Pilates
Body Power

RESHAPE YOUR BODY & TRANSFORM YOUR LIFE

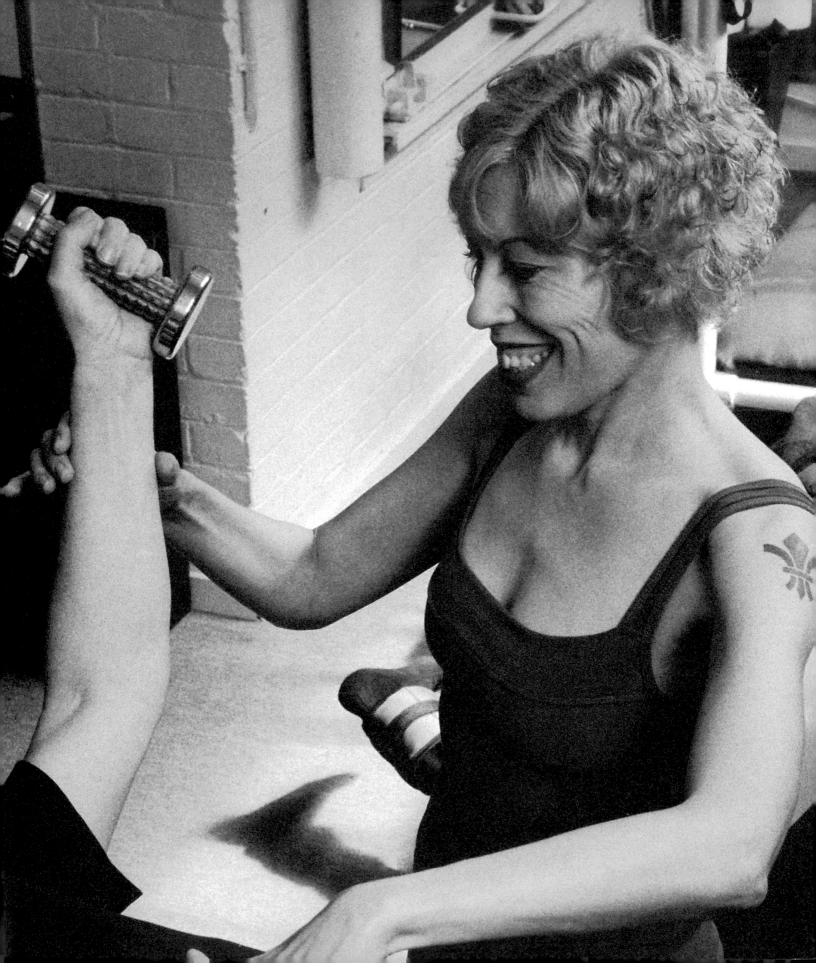

Pilates
Body Power

RESHAPE YOUR BODY & TRANSFORM YOUR LIFE

LESLEY ACKLAND

Thorsons

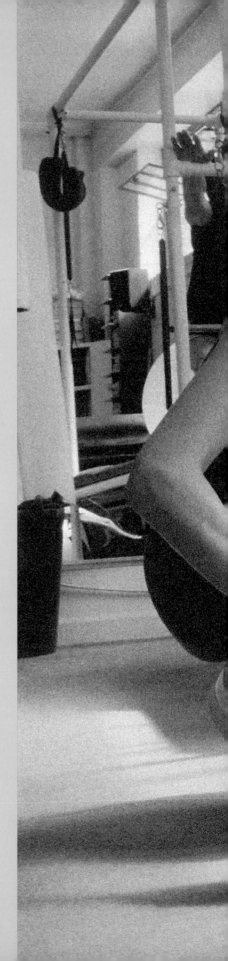

Thorsons
An Imprint of HarperCollins*Publishers*
77–85 Fulham Palace Road,
Hammersmith, London W6 8JB

The Thorsons website address is:
www.thorsons.com

Published by Thorsons 2001
10 9 8 7 6 5 4 3 2 1

Text derived from *15-Minute Pilates* and *10-step Pilates*,
published by Thorsons

Editor: Miriam Sharland
Designer: Liz Hallam
Production: Melanie Vandevelde
Index: Linda Hardcastle
Photographs by Guy Hearn

A catalogue record for this book
is available from the British Library

ISBN 0007106971

Printed in Hong Kong

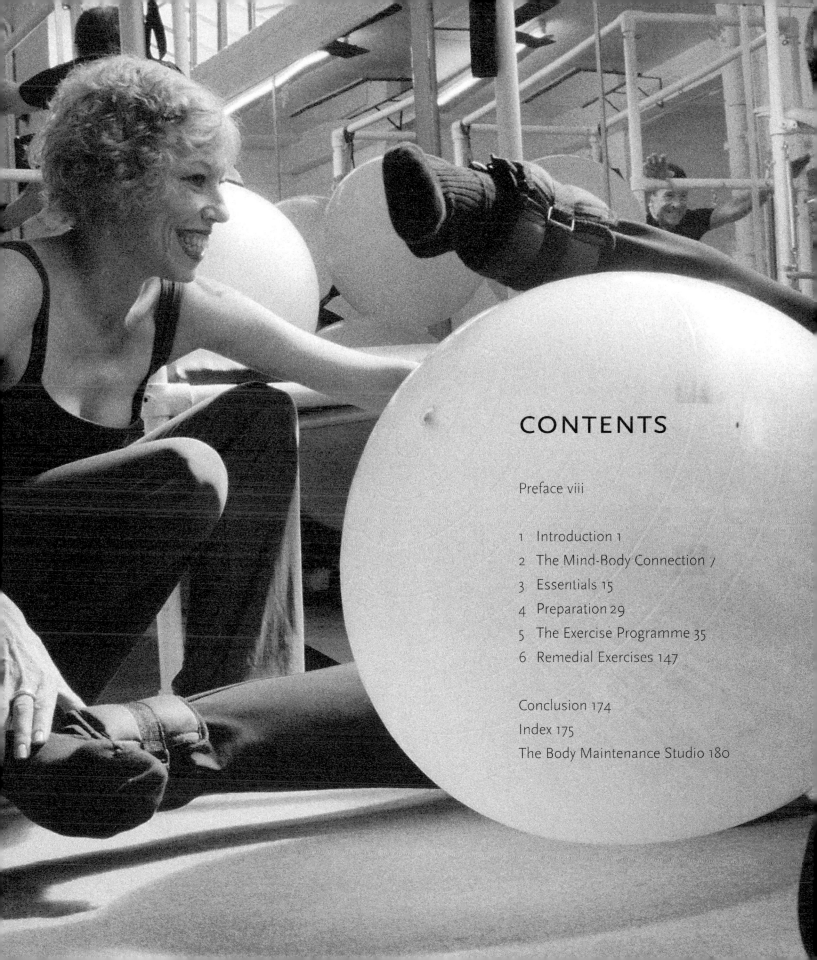

CONTENTS

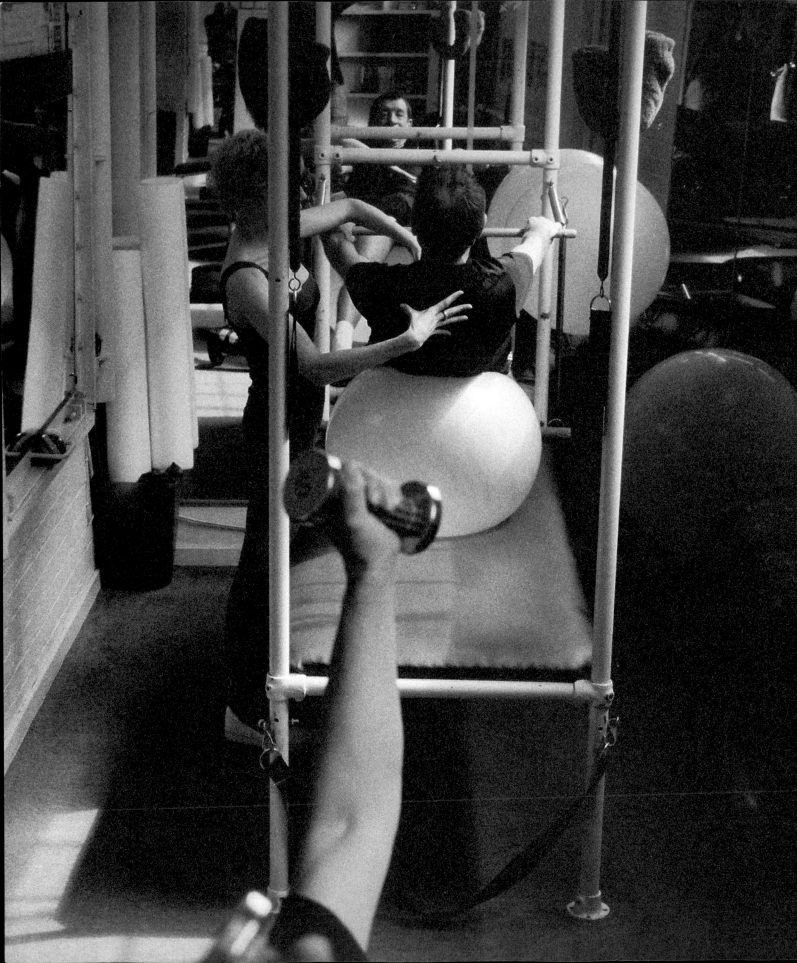

DEDICATION
To a special person, Thomas Paton

My thanks go to Janet Fitch, Caroline Hunter, Nicholas
and Yukari Ringham, Iain and Katherine Scott and Robyn
Stuart Dick. Clothing was by Bloc, Drury Lane, London
and hair was by David at Andrew Jose.

PREFACE – HOW TO USE THIS BOOK

Do you dream of a flat stomach, a longer, leaner body and superb posture? Do you wish to improve your overall appearance? If so, then *Body Power* will help you achieve all this – and more. In this book you will discover a unique bodywork system that will help you transform your body and develop a physical presence and energy that exude total confidence and grace. If you want to become healthier, stronger, leaner and more supple, my Pilates®-based Body Maintenance techniques are designed to work for all ages and all levels of fitness. There are also specific remedial techniques you can try if you suffer from medical conditions such as a bad back, scoliosis, repetitive strain injury (carpal tunnel syndrome) or sciatica.

While most people have heard of Pilates®, few know exactly what it entails. Pilates® is a very disciplined, focused form of exercise, designed to strengthen ligaments and joints, increase flexibility and lengthen the muscles. The main emphasis is on 'elongating' the body to create a longer, leaner and taller silhouette. However, Pilates® differs from other exercise regimes by going beyond the purely physical. This is a holistic discipline that integrates the mind, body and spirit. It is a philosophy of movement that brings about mental and physical integration. My Body Maintenance system of exercises is a unique system developed from Pilates® exercises.

If you have never tried this type of exercise before, you will be surprised by its apparent simplicity. The slow, controlled movements enable energy to move more freely throughout the body. The visualization techniques gently help to focus the mind so that each exercise is executed with ultimate precision. With my Pilates®-based exercises there is no need for over-exertion. The emphasis is on quality, not quantity. It's not about how much you do but, rather, how you do it. This is good news indeed for those of you who have become disillusioned and bored with fitness programmes that may not suit you.

If you want to have a long, lean look, with a minimum of effort in the safest way, you merely have to follow the guidelines in this book. Most of the techniques are based on the idea of using your own body to create resistance, so there is no need for any complicated props. All you need is a willing body and a curious mind. Before you attempt any of the exercises though, it is important that you first become acquainted with the underlying principles.

In the Introduction I outline the origins of Pilates®, and how I have evolved and updated this classic regime to make it more contemporary and accessible. Chapter 2 explains how much easier it is to bring about physical changes when you learn to focus your mind and practise visualization techniques as well.

Chapter 3 covers the basic principles of Body Maintenance, such as the importance of proper breathing, alignment and movement control. It introduces the key terms that are used throughout the book, and explains the physiological effects of Body Maintenance

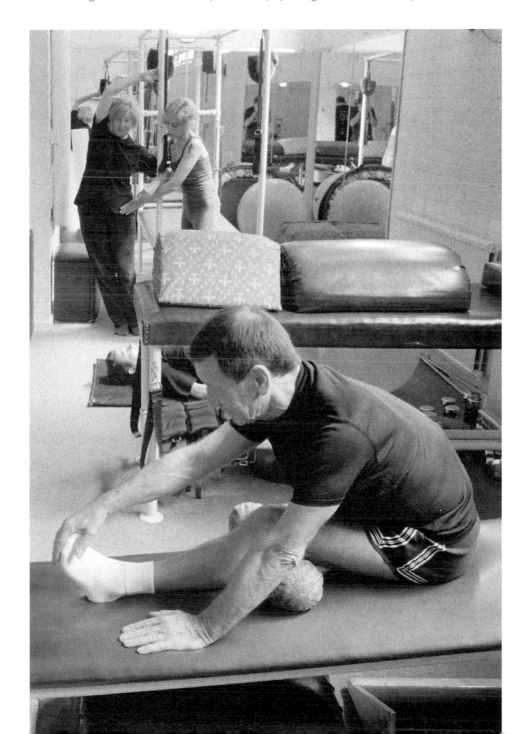

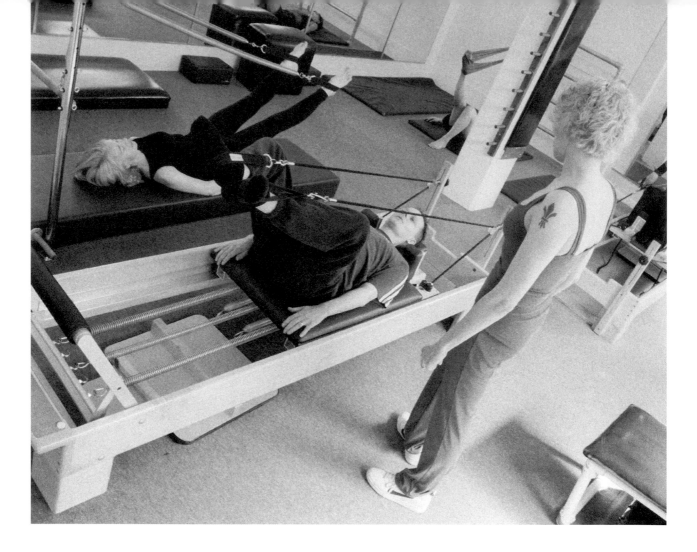

techniques on your body. For practical advice on clothes, safety, equipment and which exercises you should do, turn to Chapter 4.

The core exercise programme is outlined in Chapter 5. Here, you will find all the different types of exercise you can do, at home, every day. They include exercises to tone and strengthen your abdominal muscles, the muscles in your back, your upper body (arms, chest and shoulders) and your lower body (legs, hips and thighs), as well as a series of all the essential stretches.

If you suffer from a bad back, scoliosis, repetitive strain injury (carpal tunnel syndrome) or sciatica, you will find the relevant remedial exercises in Chapter 6.

Body Power promises no quick fixes or sudden improvements. However, with concentration and commitment, the end result will be rewarding and nothing short of enhanced physical and mental well-being.

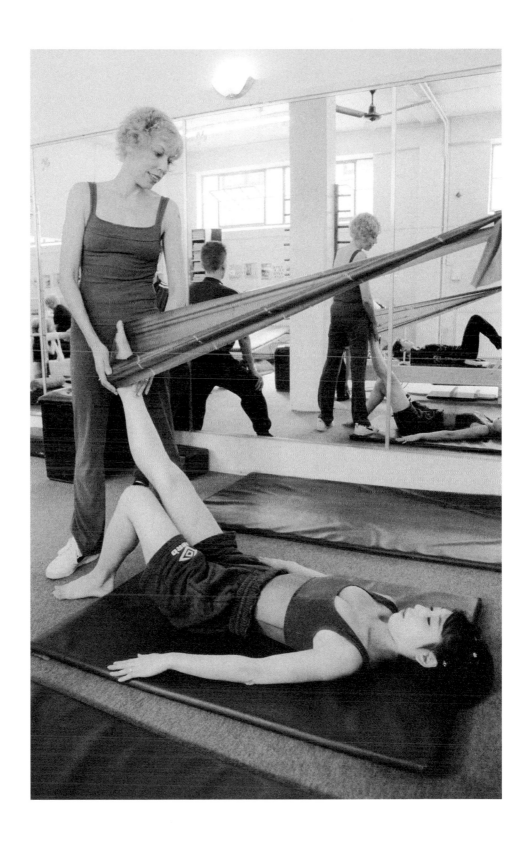

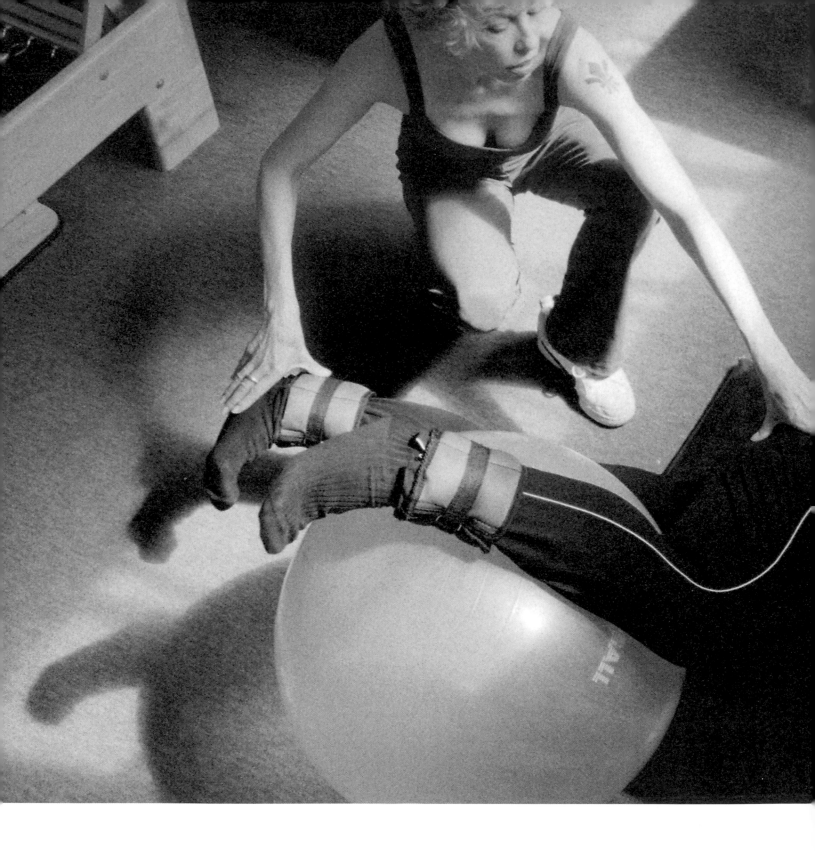

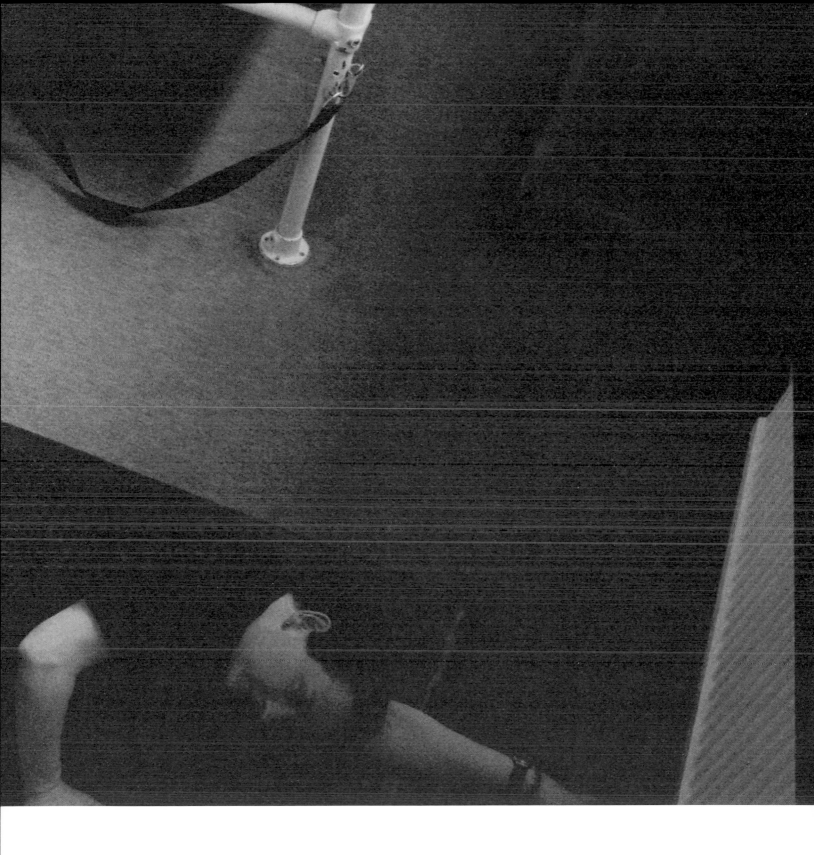

1 introduction

With Body Maintenance I believe that you can achieve the body you want in a controlled, progressive and intelligent way. Body Maintenance doesn't build bulk, but strengthens weak muscles and stretches tight ones. You can concentrate on one part of the body without straining another. Body Maintenance differs from other forms of exercise because it initially focuses on posture. Good posture is essential in realigning the body, which can have you looking and feeling taller, slimmer and well-toned.

The beauty of Body Maintenance is that it is suitable for people of all ages. Notwithstanding your level of fitness, you have the potential for achieving a supple body and reaching a level of 'wellness' that you will want to maintain. You should feel good about yourself, which involves an intelligent dialogue between your body and mind. Imagery and visualization are very appropriate tools – if you can focus on how you wish to look, the body will most assuredly co-operate. How you picture yourself is reflected in your body language which, in turn, is observed by the world at large. When that language is fluent and flowing you will be aware of it – others will comment on how well you look.

Many people do not have a positive body self-image. Women, specifically, have a tendency to retreat from their bodies as they get older. *Body Power* can help you achieve the body that you want, and are comfortable with, not the body someone else has judged to be more acceptable. Too often we are held hostage to figures in glossy magazines, imagining them to be preferable and easily attainable. I find this unrealistic, even dangerous. We should acknowledge and appreciate our own bodies and work with what we are naturally given. Many people do not even consider the highly desirable aspects of themselves. In this 'media-friendly' generation we are almost brainwashed into acknowledging 'the perfect body' hype, which is, in fact, merely the fashion of the moment. This can result in feelings of dissatisfaction and depression. We have the ability to transform ourselves, to reduce our self-imposed limitations and tap into our potential – using my techniques on a daily basis will stretch both the mind and the body.

Very few of us are born with an anatomically perfect body. Through habitual misuse, which begins when we are quite young and continues until we feel discomfort, we can seriously damage parts of the body. Unknowingly, certain areas are accentuated and, as we get older, it is more than likely that one side of the spine will be visibly over-developed. This is when problems manifest themselves. My Pilates®-based exercise programme attempts to create the best body that is possible for you, on your frame, with the understanding that there is no such thing as the perfect body. All of us have imbalances. The trouble begins when an imbalance turns into a physical problem.

For those who have repetitive strain injury (carpal tunnel syndrome), scoliosis or a myriad other problems, *Body Power* is a superb tool to use as you begin the journey towards helping and even reversing your condition. I believe that everyone can and will improve and even overcome their physical liabilities, with a safe and gentle group of exercises. You will be amazed at the body's ability to respond and rejuvenate given the correct impetus. For those of you with serious postural problems involving balance, these exercises can change not only your body, but the perception of vulnerability you feel and transmit to others. You will regain your confidence and not live in fear of falling, stumbling and giving the impression of vulnerability to others who could cause you injury.

I have never met anyone I could not help with Body Maintenance. We should not tolerate a life that is limited due to 'the back', 'the leg', etc. To embrace such negative thinking is to resign oneself to a very unsatisfactory existence and lifestyle. As you begin the following exercises be patient but determined, and feel the body working towards what you have always envisioned – the elegance of a swan's neck, the supple back of a ballet dancer. Feel yourself floating, soaring as you go through your movements. Concentrate on the moment; eventually all will be remembered as you progress. Even those of you who are extremely unfit can look forward to the day you can look in the mirror and not recognize your former selves.

THE ORIGINS OF CLASSIC PILATES®

The original concept of Pilates® was the brainchild of a German, Joseph Hubertus Pilates. He was extremely frail and weak as a child, but was determined to regain good health. This was the start of a life-long obsession with fitness and body building, and as a young man he excelled as a diver, skier and professional gymnast. At the age of 32 he moved to England, where he made a living as a boxer, circus performer and self-defence instructor.

When the First World War broke out, his career was temporarily cut short. As a German, Pilates was interned in England for the duration of the war. He used this time, however, as an opportunity to re-think and develop his approach to fitness. The result was the first blueprint for a whole new regime, Pilates, which drew upon all the various disciplines with which he was involved. His basic philosophy concluded that the only way to achieve true fitness was through the integration of mind and body. Hence, all his techniques were based on a combination of physical and mental conditioning.

When Joseph Pilates created his unique system of exercise during the early part of the twentieth century, the lifestyle was, in many respects, healthier for the public at large. Without the profusion of cars and mass transportation, walking was not merely a preferred form of exercise but, rather, the most efficient way of getting from place to place.

Many of the injuries and disabilities of today are, in fact, caused by our very modern, machine-oriented society. Repetitive movements on computers and sitting in an office chair for the greater part of the day contradict the physiological needs of the human body. There are also, of course, factors beyond our control, such as genetic traits and unfortunate injuries, which must also be addressed. I knew that I had to expand and enhance the basic principles of Pilates®.

BODY MAINTENANCE

Almost 90 years after Pilates® was created, physical ailments have changed, but pain has not. Contemporary stress has induced a variety of debilitating afflictions. In 1980 I began developing Body Maintenance, a balanced system of exercise, body shaping and toning combined with mental improvement and nutrition, based on Pilates®. I initially studied with Alan Herdman, who first brought Pilates® to the UK. Then I began travelling regularly to New York City to study Pilates® there. During my instruction abroad I became aware of a new wave of research on the human body, and I found myself looking at the way physiotherapists were working, particularly at the New York City Ballet. I had also become aware of other forms of bodywork, including Feldenkreis and the Alexander Technique.

With Pilates® as the main base, I began to integrate methods from a wide variety of sources, including remedial massage, osteopathy and injury clinics, and created my own unique system of bodywork, which I call Body Maintenance. Over the last 12 years in my own studio at Pineapple Dance Studios in London's Covent Garden, I have worked successfully with people who have suffered from a variety of modern infirmities: RSI (carpal tunnel syndrome), chronic back pain (some of which stems from spinal surgery), HIV-related problems, aerobic sprains, extreme obesity, even low self-esteem.

Often called 'yoga with machines', the Pilates®-based exercises in my studio can incorporate balls, ropes, springs and pulleys. However, the most important and long-lasting work takes place on the floor. Mat exercises, essential to body mobility and endurance, target weak, under-utilized muscles in the abdomen, lower back, arms and legs. Based on mat work, the exercises in this book are straightforward, concentrated movements that don't require a gym or special equipment. What they do require are a few minutes – in the morning, during lunch, or later in the evening. This is a complete exercise regime devised for individuals who might not have the inclination or opportunity to seek out my studio, but who want to benefit from my tried and proven Pilates®-based Body Maintenance programme.

For those of you who wish to enhance or change some aspect of your bodies, this routine is simple and straightforward. People tend to use their big muscles for everything. I work on strengthening the smaller muscles, which can give you the shape that you want. You can tone your stomach, thighs and arms and reshape your buttocks as well. Get into swimsuit shape – look and feel longer, leaner and more glamorous. There is no limit to what you can expect to achieve. My workout will have you feeling supple, slender and self-assured. Your entire view of yourself, both physically and emotionally, will improve and you will reach that summit of 'wellness' where the mind-body-spirit positively connect. The rest is up to you.

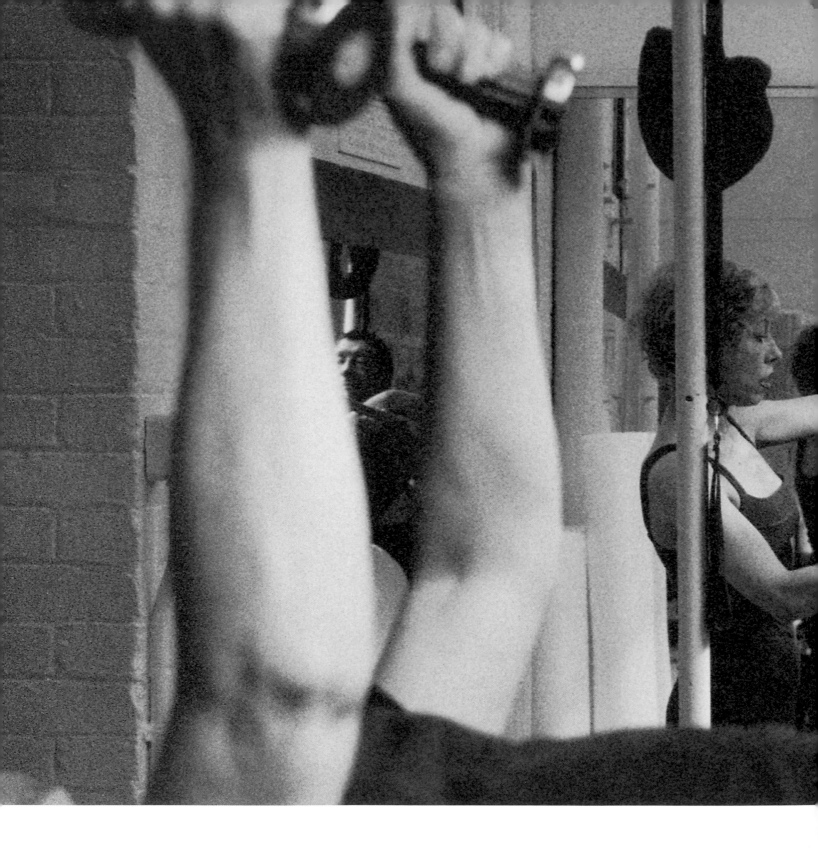

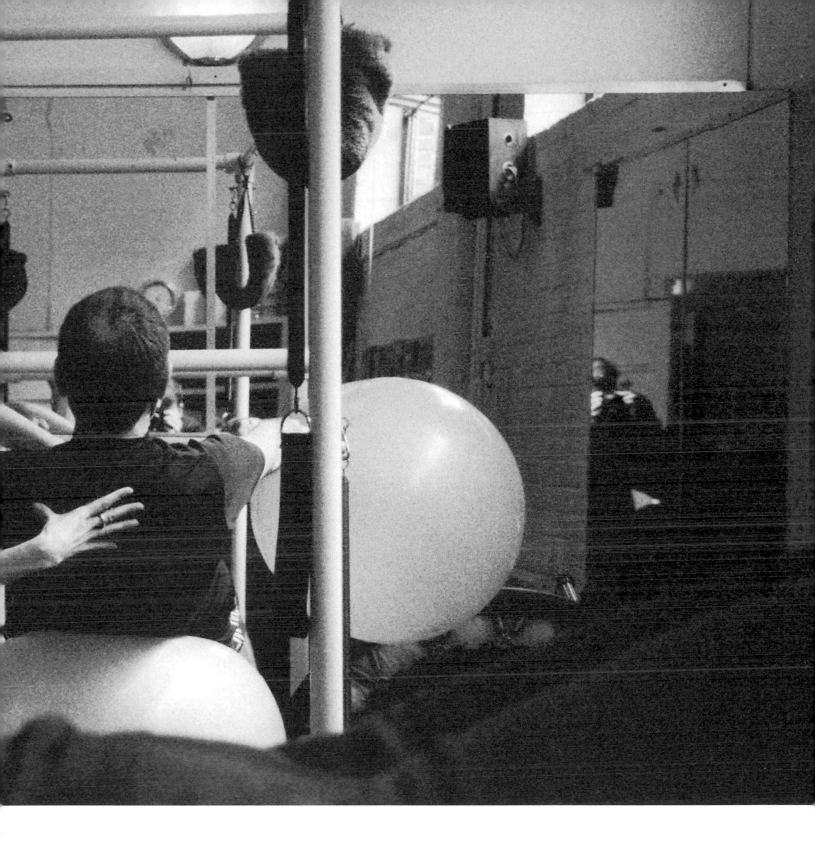

2 the mind–body connection

The main principle of Body Maintenance is that exercise is essentially a mind–body technique. Therefore, when you exercise you should mentally focus on the muscle groups that you are using. Body Maintenance recognizes that it is only through the synchronizing of thought and action that an exercise is truly effective. In order to create a healthy and fit body you need to integrate the mental, physical and spiritual spheres.

MIND OVER MATTER

It has long been established that the mind has an enormous influence on the health of the body. Research shows that the mind has an infinite capacity to induce positive physiological effects, which have both an internal and external effect. You may have noticed that when you're in a good mood you automatically seem to look and feel better. Scientists ascribe this phenomenon to the activity of the billions of nerve cells in our brain, which transmit chemical messages to the rest of the body. Our thoughts and emotions play a vital role in influencing this intercellular communication.

Think for a moment how you feel when you are stressed. Not very pleasant. This is because your body produces an excess of 'stress' chemicals (e.g. adrenaline and cortisol) which causes your whole system to speed up. Your heart beats faster, your blood pressure goes up, your breathing becomes rapid and shallow. At times, this type of response is necessary. It is what motivates you when you are faced with a crisis. In large doses this type of reaction can, however, be extremely harmful and lead to all sorts of unpleasant symptoms such as dizziness, shaking, profuse sweating, insomnia and migraines. It is easy to see what effect negative, stress-inducing emotions can have.

Positive feelings of calm and contentment have a much more beneficial effect, as they induce the body to produce health-enhancing, feel-good chemicals (e.g. endorphins and serotonin), which are vital for well-being. They promote a sense of serenity – you breathe more easily and deeply, your heart rate is slower and your blood pressure lowers. The more relaxed you feel, the less tension you hold in the muscles throughout your body. This has a beneficial effect on your general bearing and posture. Tight, tense muscles make your body shrink and constrict. This stops the energy from flowing freely throughout the body and, in time, this will be reflected in a weak, misshapen musculature.

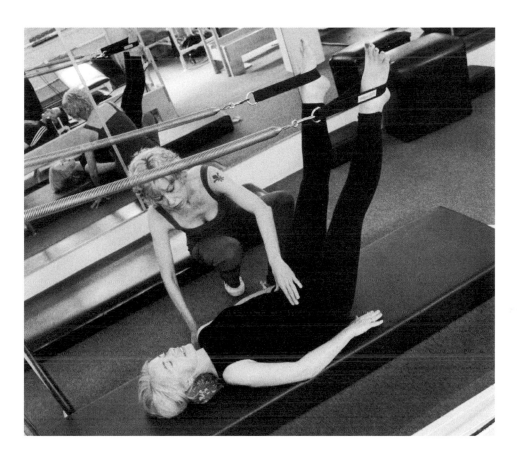

MINDFUL EXERCISE

If thoughts are so powerful, it makes sense to try and harness your thinking to bring about positive changes in your body. This is, in fact, the very essence of Body Maintenance. By learning to execute each exercise correctly you are also allowing your mind to exert a greater influence over your body. With Body Maintenance you only do a limited number of repetitions. You do them slowly, so that you can concentrate more clearly on directing your energy towards what it is that you are trying to achieve. If you view your body in a negative way you will need to reverse your direction of thought. Positive thoughts bring about positive changes.

To ensure that an exercise is of real benefit and will bring about the changes that you desire – for example a strong, straight back – it is necessary to complement each physical action with a mental focus. By practising creative visualization regularly, you will gradually develop the intellectual and emotional ability to internalize the physical changes you wish to make. Once you've done this, the external changes will start to appear.

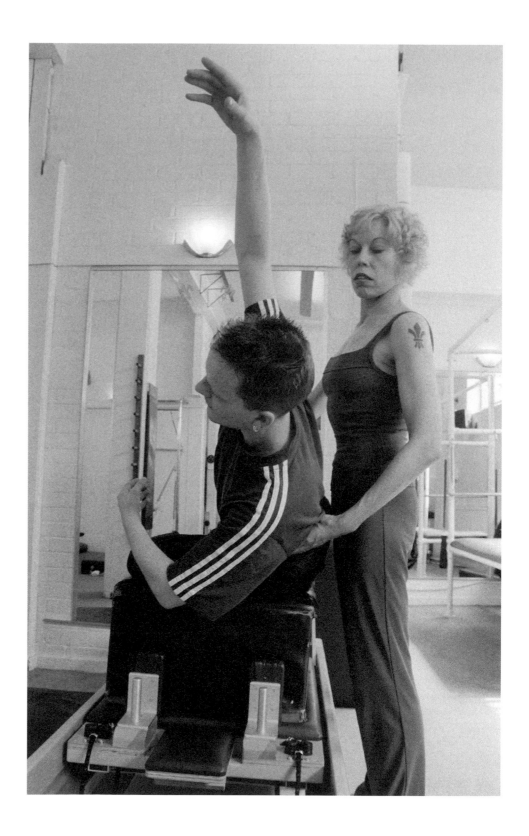

As you become aware of your body and its needs, you can consciously start to make changes through exercise. Body Maintenance is based on lengthening and stretching the body to its full potential. This eventually creates a longer, leaner shape, increased flexibility and a suppleness that promotes a greater ease of movement. These exercises concentrate on strengthening weak muscles and stretching those that are too tight and constricted. What you really want is a body in which strength and flexibility complement each other. It is possible to totally re-structure the way you are. It is not, however, just a matter of getting your body to make the right moves. An integral part of Body Maintenance is the way you perceive the exercise. This is why attitude and creative imagery are so important. Each time you work through a series of movements it is essential that you can envision what it is that you wish to achieve. Painting a picture in your mind helps your body to respond in the right way. This not only makes the whole process more stimulating but also makes the effect of each exercise much more powerful. Initially it may take a while to fully understand the mechanisms. I always tell a new client to expect to do only about 30 per cent of what he or she will eventually be capable of doing. It takes about 10 sessions to really comprehend the technique. Body Maintenance is one of the few forms of exercise that gets progressively more difficult, but the results are worth it. In time you will look taller, slimmer and more toned.

CREATIVE VISUALIZATION

Whatever we create in our lives begins as a basic image in our minds. Many of these images are unconscious. Through creative visualization it is possible to alter these thoughts and pictures. With Body Maintenance, the idea is to create an image in your mind that will help you to focus on the area of the body that you are working. This requires a very deep level of concentration, which does become easier with practice. On a superficial level, many of the exercises appear quite simple. How you physically position your arms and legs, however, is only part of the process. Body Maintenance, unlike many other disciplines, is actually much more complex, as with each movement you must be constantly aware of what your entire body is doing. You don't concentrate only on the stomach, or the inner thigh, and exclude the rest of your body. Even when you are doing a series of movements specifically designed to work a certain group of muscles, such as your abdominals or your quads, you must always remember to be equally focused on the rest of your body. Where are your feet? Are you holding your head in exactly the right way? Is your body properly aligned?

Initially, this can seem quite difficult and using visualization techniques can be enormously helpful. By understanding how your body should be feeling it becomes easier to assume the correct position. Eventually, these images will arise naturally through association, without too much effort. Visualization is one of the best methods to bridge the gap between mind and body. By creating mental pictures that correspond to what you are trying to do physically you will, in time, develop a level of body awareness that is unique to Pilates®-based exercises.

Basic Visualization Techniques

Anyone can learn to visualize. It helps if you can begin by feeling relaxed. A still mind is more conducive to conjuring up images.

▷ Spend a few minutes gathering your thoughts. Try to forget about external influences such as work, what you should be doing and any worries you might have. Remember, this is your time.

▷ Do some gentle stretches and focus on your breathing. Slow, deep breathing has an instantly calming effect because it helps to promote soothing alpha brainwaves. Once you are feeling sufficiently relaxed you can start your exercises.

▷ As you exercise, focus on each part of your body. How does it feel? With each exercise try to perceive a specific picture. If you are trying to envision yourself on a sandy beach, focus clearly on how this feels. Do your feet feel relaxed, warm and comfortable? Are your arms hanging loosely by your sides, like a puppet? Where is your head? Think of images that will help you to get into exactly the right position.

▷ Invite each image to emerge with as much intensity as possible, so that you can almost feel it. Once you have created a familiar picture, eventually all you will have to do is to focus on it and your body will automatically respond.

The aim of Body Maintenance exercises is to bring about permanent changes. You can hasten this process by using visualization techniques when you are not exercising. These will automatically help you to walk, stand and sit in the correct way.

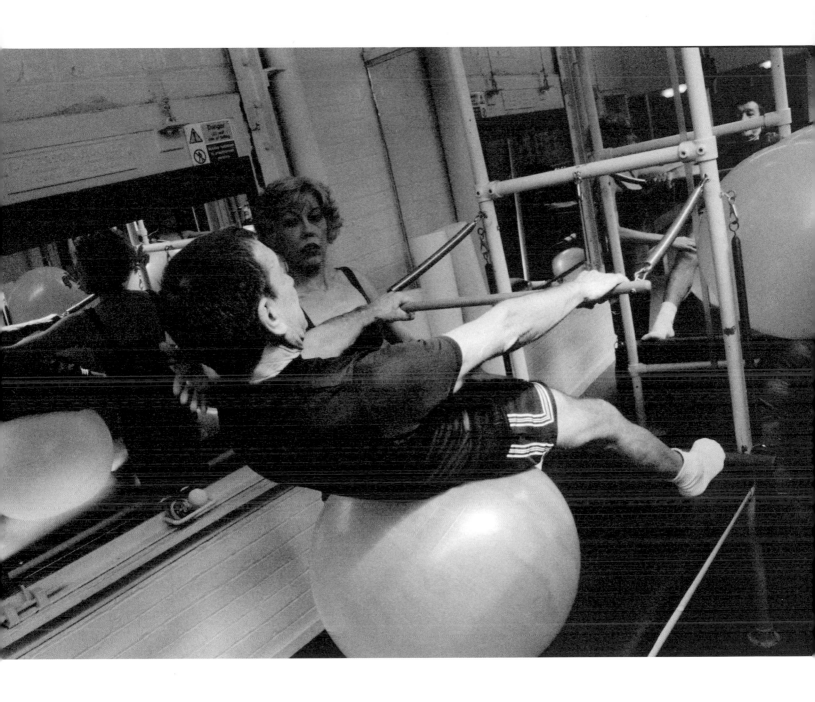

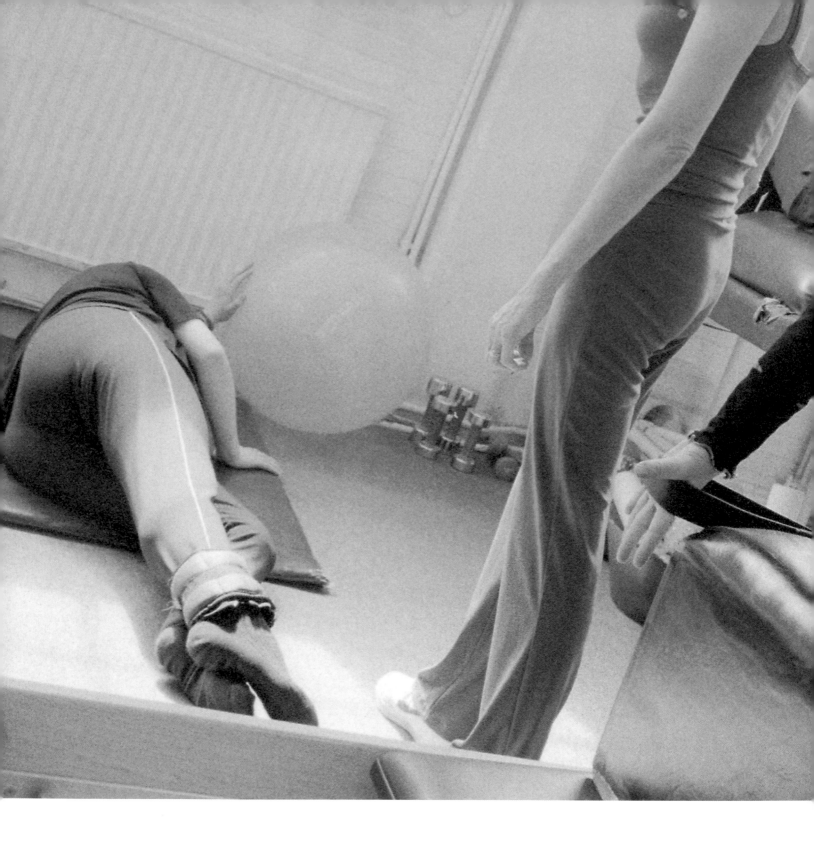

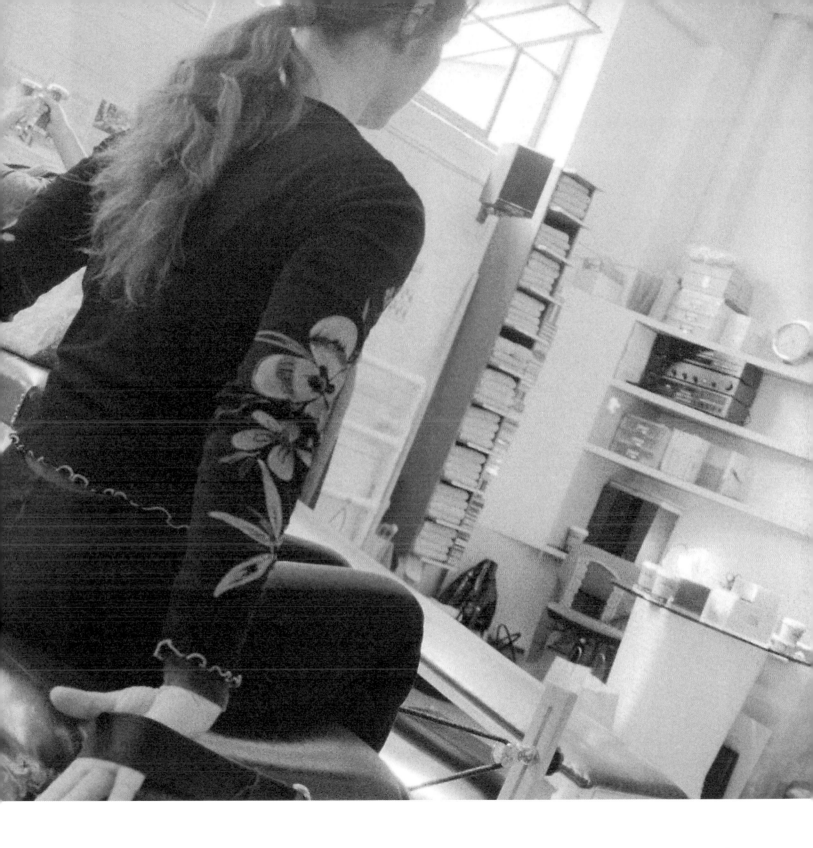

3 essentials

Pilates®-based Body Maintenance is a very precise system of exercise. It is different from other regimes in that it requires a bit of groundwork before you start. In order to understand fully what you are doing it is important that you first become acquainted with the basic principles. There are six essential guidelines to remember.

1 BREATHING

In dance a lot of emphasis is placed on the relationship between breath and movement. However, the importance of breath is a topic rarely addressed in the gym. Body Maintenance differs from conventional forms of exercise in that it concentrates on the correct use of breathing for each and every exercise.

Breath nourishes the body and the brain. People tend to breathe shallowly into their upper bodies when they inhale, into the upper chest and not right down into their lower lobes. If you are breathing deeply, you're working from the inside out. You are energizing and replenishing large areas of your body. Again, it is as much a spiritual as a physical idea.

For most of the exercises in this book, you will breathe out on the point of effort. During the exercises think about oxygen as a rejuvenating life-force. Always exhale on the point of effort. If you have a tight area, try and breathe into that – breath is another form of liberation, working from the inside out.

Most people are stronger on one side than on the other, looser on one side and tighter on the other. You are using exercise and breath to create equilibrium in the body.

2 CONTROL

All the exercises in *Body Power* are controlled. In this particular instance the word 'controlled' means that the correct body parts are being used. Many people, for example, thinking that they are using their abdominals during an exercise, are, in fact using their bones or hip flexors. Thus, the muscles that should be targeted are not being worked in an efficient way.

Control and precision go together. All these exercises are done slowly, in a meditative fashion. You focus the mind on what you're doing, and don't allow it to wander. You use breath, coordination, control and precision to do a limited number of repetitions well.

You minimize the stress and involvement of other parts of the body. It's preferable to do even five repetitions in a slow and regulated way, than to go through hundreds of motions, during which time nothing effective has happened. In the pelvic tilts, you should be able to feel, literally, one vertebra at a time. The fact that you do 10 repetitions in Body Maintenance well is better than doing many repetitions badly.

The same principle applies when you are using free-standing weights. In this case, you should be thinking about using internal resistance rather than using your shoulders or snapping your elbows as you use the weights. Focus on the muscles you're using, while making sure that the rest of the body is relaxed and aligned. People often make what is a simple exercise into something quite tortuous, thus creating distortion, tension and the inability to minimize the movements of other parts of their bodies.

3 CENTRING

In many Eastern religions, the centre of the body is not the heart, but the pelvis. The main principle of the Body Maintenance technique is to recognize that there is one strong, core area that controls the rest of the body. This is located in that part of your body that forms a continuous band at the back and front, between the bottom of your rib-cage and across the line of your hipbones. This is called the centre. This is the area in which the muscles in your stomach and back are – at the centre of your body. These muscles support the internal organs and keep you upright. If you have a strong centre you have a strong back, which means you can walk, stand and run without discomfort or pain. Your arms and legs are extensions of this part of your body. If you have a bad back this is an indication that the centre is not strong enough. Originally human beings were not designed to stand upright. The only reason we stand at all is due to these specific muscles. We are constantly fighting gravity, which pulls us forward. This explains why so many people have all sorts of problems with those muscles affiliated with the shoulders and neck. We are basically defying nature, gravity and our initial body type.

4 FLOW

Each movement in Body Maintenance is designed to be performed in a smooth, flowing, undulating way. There is no room within this regime for any sharp, jarring movements or quick, jerky actions – these are the total antithesis of everything you are trying to achieve. If a movement ever feels like this, you can be sure that you are doing it wrong. Every motion originates from a strong centre and flows in a slow, gentle, controlled fashion, thus warming the muscles and causing them to lengthen and open up the spaces between each vertebra in the spine so that the body expands to create a longer, leaner shape.

5 PRECISION

In order to be effective, all Pilates®-based exercises have to be performed with exact precision. This attention to detail is important as it ensures that each movement is working the body in the correct manner. Before you start an exercise sequence, read the instructions carefully. Pay full attention to proper alignment and check what the 'watchpoints' have to say. This will ensure that you do not expend excess energy doing an exercise incorrectly.

6 COORDINATION

Children run naturally, but for most adults basic coordination is a major problem. Many people, when starting Body Maintenance complain to me, 'I can't coordinate my breath and the movement. It's too much. I've got to concentrate too hard. I can't do it.' Most of us have lost the ability to coordinate the mind and body into a working machine. We no longer have the sense of our feet being in contact with the earth. We've lost the feeling of the way the breath moves naturally through the body. The aim is to retrain the neuromuscular connection between the brain and the body.

This is best illustrated when I try and teach foot exercises to people. I sometimes joke that the feet are very far from the brain and they won't obey, as they haven't been asked to do anything for a long time. Observe people who have lost the use of their hands. They can do the same things with their feet that others can do with their hands. We all have that capability, but we don't employ it. If you don't avail yourself of something it atrophies. Therefore, if you don't use coordination in the physical sense you lose the ability.

Some of the exercises in *Body Power* appear quite complicated; that's because they're based upon the introduction of a more complicated concept than mere physical movement. They are trying to reintroduce the mind to the mind/body equation. If I ask my opposite arm and leg to do something at the same time, coordinating from the breath and a strong centre, I should be able to achieve it. If I slip in the street, I am more likely to regain my balance than not. If someone throws a bunch of keys at me, I will probably be able to catch it. Because I have the neuromuscular connection between the mind and body parts, I can be spontaneous, and this is where the proprioceptive concept – the linking of mind and body – comes into play.

In *Body Power*, we try to re-create your body as a coordinated whole, rather than thinking 'I am exercising an arm or leg or the stomach.' Coordination is paramount to the way the exercises flow. You might see a Body Maintenance exercise that is similar to those used in aerobic classes or at a gym, but the difference between a Body Maintenance exercise and an aerobic one is that, in Body Maintenance, the movement is concentrated exercise and requires minimal effort from other parts of the body.

KEY TERMS

In Pilates® and Body Maintenance there are certain key terms that are referred to over and over again. It helps if you understand these before you begin.

Relaxing

Pilates® frequently refers to keeping an area relaxed. This isn't necessarily what you might think. Most people associate relaxation with a feeling of 'letting go', of allowing muscles to slump. In this case, to relax means to release tension in an area while still managing to maintain tone and control. This should feel comfortable and natural.

Neutral Spine

Some of the positions you will be assuming require your spine to remain in neutral. This means that you maintain the natural curve in your back. Thus, when you are lying down, do not press your back so hard into the floor that you lose your natural curve. Neither must you allow your back to arch so that your lower back comes off the floor. Just lie there, breathe in and out naturally and allow your back to relax into the floor without pressing it in. This will permit your back to relax into its natural, neutral position – which is slightly different for everybody.

The Centre

With Body Maintenance, every exercise originates from the centre. The stomach muscles are the core to everything and support the spine. It is important that you always remember to keep this area correctly aligned. This is particularly important when you exercise the lower abdominals as it is very easy to do the opposite of what you actually want. It is natural when you breathe in for the stomach to pull into the spine and when you breathe out for it to bulge. This is not what you want. You will have to try and reverse what the body wants to do unconsciously. As you breathe in you should relax the stomach; as you breathe out you should pull the navel to the spine, engaging the lower abdominal muscles. Your body will naturally want to do the opposite, but it's important to engage the stomach muscles when you exhale.

The Feet

The main thing to remember when exercising is that most of the time you want your feet to be relaxed. If you are in doubt – relax your feet. Most people tense their feet too much and as a result constantly complain about getting cramp in their feet when they are exercising. (If you do get cramp use a foot roller to ease away the tension.) A relaxed foot should feel comfortable, so that there is no sensation of tightness. Whenever you are required to flex your feet, do so by gently stretching out your heel then pulling the top of your foot as far as you can without straining. Do not tense your foot so that it feels strained.

The Neck

This is a sensitive part of the body, so you do not want to put it under unnecessary strain while you are exercising. It is very important that you always follow the neck instructions very carefully. Body Maintenance often refers to keeping your neck long, which means adjusting your head into a position that lengthens your neck. When you are doing an exercise lying on your back, the way you bring your head into alignment with the rest of your body is by moving the top of your skull and the base of your neck. Do not attempt to flatten your neck against the floor.

Straight Arms and Legs

This is a very common term in Body Maintenance. Your arms and legs should be relaxed and not locked. This is an important point to remember, particularly for the stretches. If an exercise requires that you stretch your arm or leg out straight, you should take care not to overextend, which causes the joints to lock.

BODY BASICS

The main function of the skeletal system is to provide your body with support, protection and movement. Bones act as levers and when muscles pull on the bones, this causes parts of the body to move. Muscles are attached to the bones by tendons composed of tough, fibrous, non-elastic connective tissue. The bones you should be most concerned about in Body Maintenance are the main 25 bones that comprise the spinal column, consisting of:

▷ seven cervical vertebrae in the neck
▷ twelve thoracic vertebrae articulating with the ribs in the thorax
▷ five lumbar vertebrae in the lower back
▷ four bones fused together into the coccyx at the base of the spine.

One Vertebra at a Time

Body Maintenance frequently refers to the term one vertebra at a time. This is one of the main principles that you should keep in mind whenever you are doing an exercise that involves rolling your body up from and down to the mat. The idea is that you always roll up gradually so that you are lifting only one vertebra off the mat at a time. The same rule applies when you roll back down again. This takes some practice and initially you will need to concentrate very carefully to ensure that you are doing it correctly.

Movements

All movements involving the bones occur at the joints, thus enabling a variety of different movements. The more common ones that you are likely to come across in Body Maintenance include:

FLEXION – which bends a limb or the spine, e.g. when bending the head forward onto the chest.

EXTENSION – which straightens a limb or the spine.

HYPEREXTENSION – which means bending back further than the vertical position, e.g. moving the head backwards to look up at the ceiling.

ABDUCTION – when you make a move away from the centre of the body, e.g. raising your arms horizontally sideways.

ADDUCTION – when you move towards the centre of the body, e.g. you lower your arms to the sides.

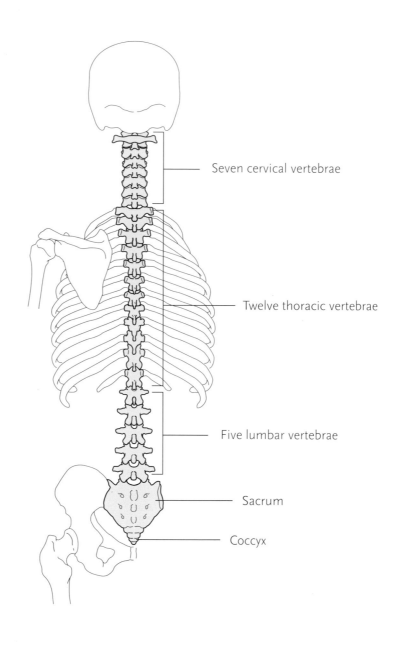

Seven cervical vertebrae

Twelve thoracic vertebrae

Five lumbar vertebrae

Sacrum

Coccyx

INVERSION – when something turns inwards, e.g. you turn the sole of your foot inwards.

ROTATION – when the bone turns on its axis either away from or towards the centre of the body.

The Muscles

Muscles create a movement by exerting a pull on the tendons, which move the bones at the joints. They are also responsible for maintaining posture. Many muscles are attached by the tendons to two articulating bones. Most movements, therefore, involve the use of several muscle groups. Muscles may also work in 'antagonistic' pairs – one muscle contracts to move the bone in one direction; the other muscle contracts to move it back, e.g. the calf and shin muscles which raise and lower the foot. Each muscle has the ability to contract or shorten. It can be stretched when it is relaxed. Muscles also control internal functions such as pumping blood round the body and the propulsion of food through the digestive system. There are literally hundreds of muscles in the body (there are 620 muscles that can be consciously controlled alone), all of which are involved in a wide range of functions.

The most important muscles you should be aware of for the purposes of Body Maintenance are:

TRAPEZIUS – in the back of the neck running down to the shoulders.
Action – extends the head.

LEVATOR SCAPULAE – at the back and sides of the neck, running into the shoulder.
Action – lifts the shoulder blade and shoulder.

DELTOID – on top of the shoulders and upper arms.
Action – moves the arm backwards and forwards.

BICEPS – at the front of the arms.
Action – moves the arm.

TRICEPS – at the back of the arm.
Action – moves the arm.

GLUTEUS MAXIMUS – forms the buttocks.
Action – raises the body, used in running and jumping.

GLUTEUS MINIMUS – in the buttocks.
Action – rotates thigh laterally, maintains balance, used in walking and running.

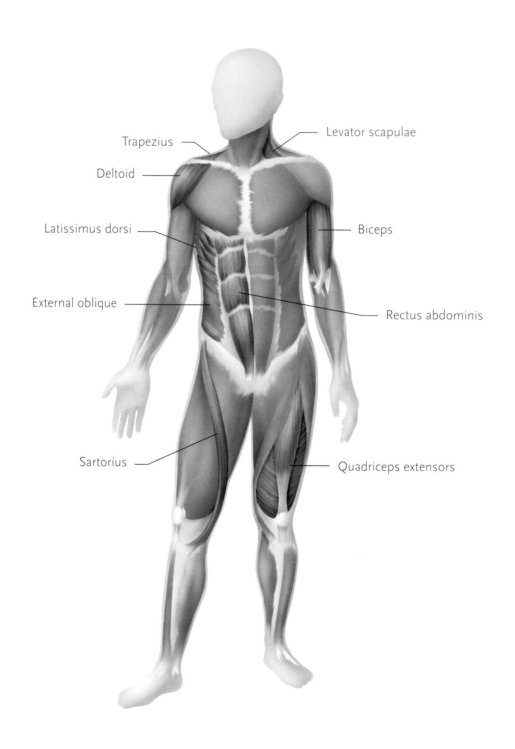

Trapezius

Deltoid

Latissimus dorsi

External oblique

Sartorius

Levator scapulae

Biceps

Rectus abdominis

Quadriceps extensors

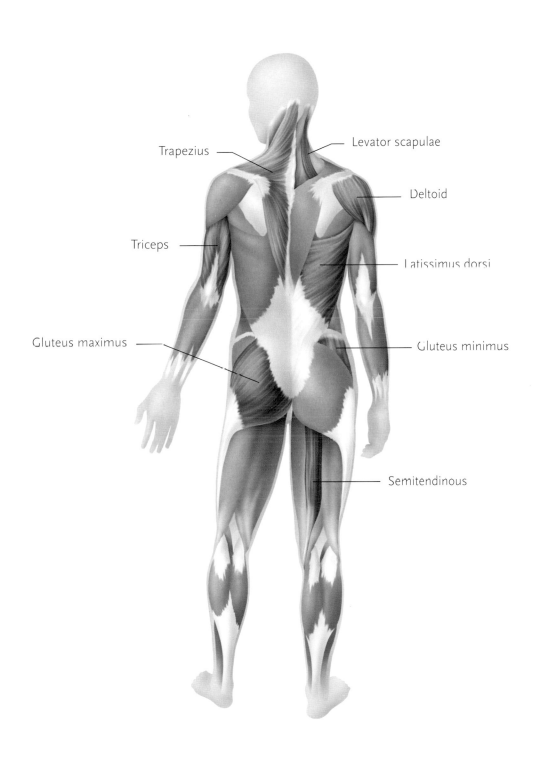

Trapezius

Levator scapulae

Deltoid

Triceps

Latissimus dorsi

Gluteus maximus

Gluteus minimus

Semitendinous

SARTORIUS – crosses front of thigh from lateral to medial side.

Action – flexes hip and knee, e.g. when sitting cross-legged.

SEMITENDINOSUS (HAMSTRINGS) – down posterior medial side of thigh.

Action – extends thigh, flexes leg at knee.

QUADRICEPS EXTENSOR – on the front of the thigh.

Action – opposite movement to hamstrings.

EXTERNAL OBLIQUE – extends laterally down the side of the abdomen.

Action – compresses abdomen, twists trunk.

INTERNAL OBLIQUE – extends laterally down the side of the front of the abdomen.

Action – compresses abdomen, twists trunk, works with the external oblique.

RECTUS ABDOMINIS – runs down the entire length of the front of the abdomen (divided into four sections).

Action – an important muscle for maintaining posture, draws front of pelvis upwards.

TRANSVERSE ABDOMINIS – runs laterally across front of abdomen.

Action – compresses abdomen.

ERECTOR SPINAE – found medially on the posterior surface of neck, thorax and abdomen.

Action – extends the spine, holds body upright.

LATISSIMUS DORSI – runs down back of lower thorax and lumbar region.

Action – draws shoulders downwards and backwards, adducts and rotates arm, helps pull body up.

BODY AWARENESS

Before you begin the Body Maintenance programme, try this simple preliminary body awareness exercise.

Standing or sitting, close your eyes. Take a few deep breaths and, starting with your head, slowly direct your focus down through your entire body. Imagine that you are steering the flow of energy throughout your body. As you do this try to visualize all the different parts of your body along the way. Think of your eyes, ears, mouth, down the shoulders, arms and hands. Visualize your chest, back, abdomen, hips, pelvic area, upper legs, knees, lower legs, ankles and feet. As you visit each area try to build up a mental picture of how it looks and feels. Spend a few seconds tuning into each part. Move your head gently, shrug your shoulders. Gently move your stomach, tailbone and hips. As you do this, concentrate on the sensation. Which areas feel most comfortable and relaxed? Are certain areas tight and constricted? Do this for a few minutes each day. This will help you to become more aware of your body when you are ready to begin the exercises.

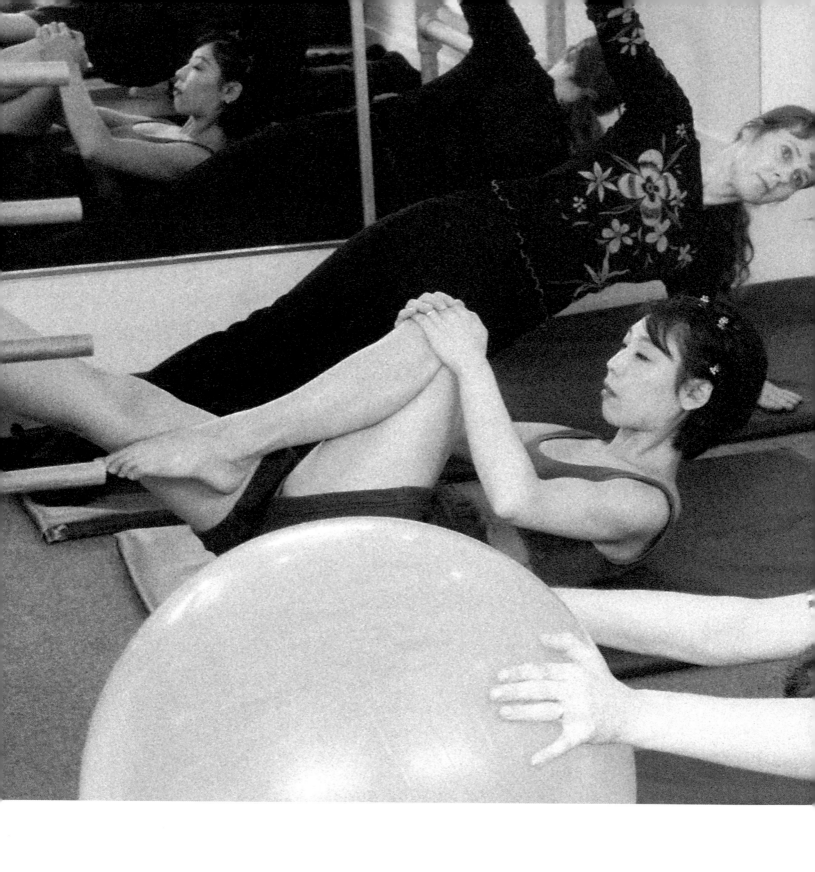

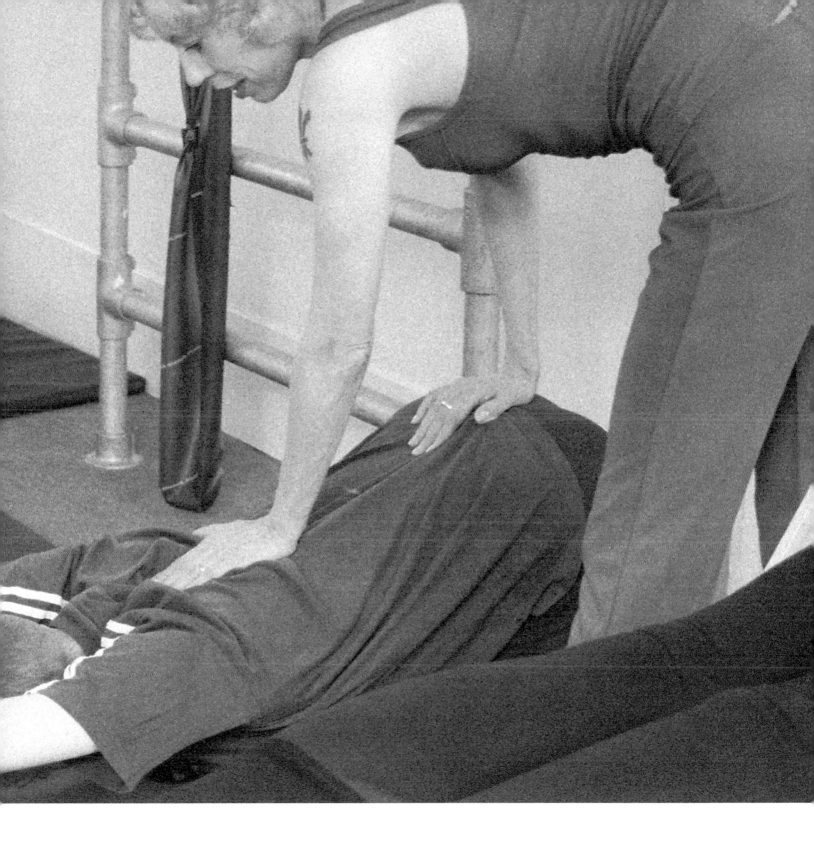

4 preparation

WHAT YOU SHOULD KNOW BEFORE YOU START TO EXERCISE

The Pilates®-based Body Maintenance exercises require total concentration and focus. This makes it particularly important to find a time and place to do them where you know you will not be disturbed. This might mean switching off the telephone and ridding yourself of other distractions so that you're not interrupted. You will also need to create a specific space for yourself where you can exercise. Most of us do not have the facilities to have our own private gyms! You may, however, find an area in your house that becomes your own retreat. It helps if you get into the right frame of mind. Do this by thinking – this is my time, I am creating a space within my house, within my environment, to work on my body for myself, without distractions.

When to Exercise

The exercises in the core exercise programme can be done at any time of the day. You might find that you prefer to do them in the early evening, to help you unwind and loosen tight muscles after a busy day. If you find it difficult to get going in the mornings, a 15-minute session first thing may be just what you need.

Clothes

Ideally, you should wear clothing in which you can exercise comfortably, such as leggings, shorts and a T-shirt, or leotard top. Don't wear anything that will restrict your movements. Opt for natural fibres like cotton, which are cooler. You can exercise wearing socks or in bare feet. If you are concerned about slipping, put on a pair of trainers. Take off any jewellery that might get in the way.

Equipment

Having picked a suitable spot in which to exercise, try to create adequate room. This may mean moving the furniture and clearing away any clutter. Before you start, check the floor for any sharp objects or stray pins. Most of the exercises require little or no equipment. It is essential however to work on a padded surface or a mat. This will protect your spine and prevent any bruising against a hard floor. It is probably worth investing in a proper sports mat. Alternatively, you can work on a folded, synthetic blanket. This should be about five or six feet long and a foot wide. Some of the exercises involve using props such as a chair, sofa, tennis ball or towel. Always make sure furniture is secure. If an exercise indicates that you need a couple of light handweights and you don't have any, you can substitute cans of beans. If possible, try exercising in front of a full-length mirror. This will enable you to check what you are doing.

WHICH EXERCISES?

With the Body Maintenance Exercise Programme it is really important to always start your core exercise routine with the pelvic tilts and the abdominal exercises, because you will be working from a strong centre. Even when working your arms and legs, everything is controlled from the centre. Thus, if you are standing and doing a calf stretch, you should be thinking about the location of your stomach, spine and shoulders. As well as doing some basic abdominal work, each session you do should also incorporate stretches after the relevant strengthening exercises. You can then do upper and lower body work on alternate days.

If you have a specific medical condition such as repetitive strain injury (carpal tunnel syndrome), scoliosis, sciatica or a bad back, only do those exercises that are recommended for that particular condition (see chapter 6).

Sequence of Exercises

1) Do all the pelvic tilt and abdominal exercises at the beginning.
2) Proceed to the back exercises.
3) Do leg exercises and stretches.
4) Finish with upper body exercises and stretches.

Read all the instructions carefully. Remember the breathing instructions.

Continue to add exercises each day as you feel more comfortable. Use your own judgement. If you are unsure do the pelvic tilts and abdominal exercises, then add to them. If you feel any discomfort in your back during any particular exercise, you still have insufficient core strength to do it.

In Body Maintenance there are a number of basic safety rules:
▷ Always do stretches after the relevant strengthening exercises.
▷ Do not attempt to do too much too soon. Increase the number of repetitions gradually.

- ▷ If you feel nauseous, fatigued or extremely breathless – stop.
- ▷ If you have any chest pains (especially when accompanied by pain in the arm, neck, shoulders and jaw) – stop exercising immediately and seek medical help.
- ▷ If exercise leaves you unnaturally tired, check with your doctor.
- ▷ The neck is a sensitive area of the body. If you cannot remember whether you have worked this area or not, it is better not to do any further repetitions.
- ▷ Always make sure that there is something you can hold on to for support when doing the balancing exercises.
- ▷ If you experience back pain – stop.
- ▷ If your muscles start shaking – stop.
- ▷ Drink plenty of fluids afterwards, especially when it is hot.

Before you embark on any new programme, it's a good idea to consult your doctor. A pre-exercise check-up is strongly advised if you are over 40 or have not been exercising regularly. Always seek the advice of a specialist if you have a medical condition, are pregnant or have any chronic joint problems.

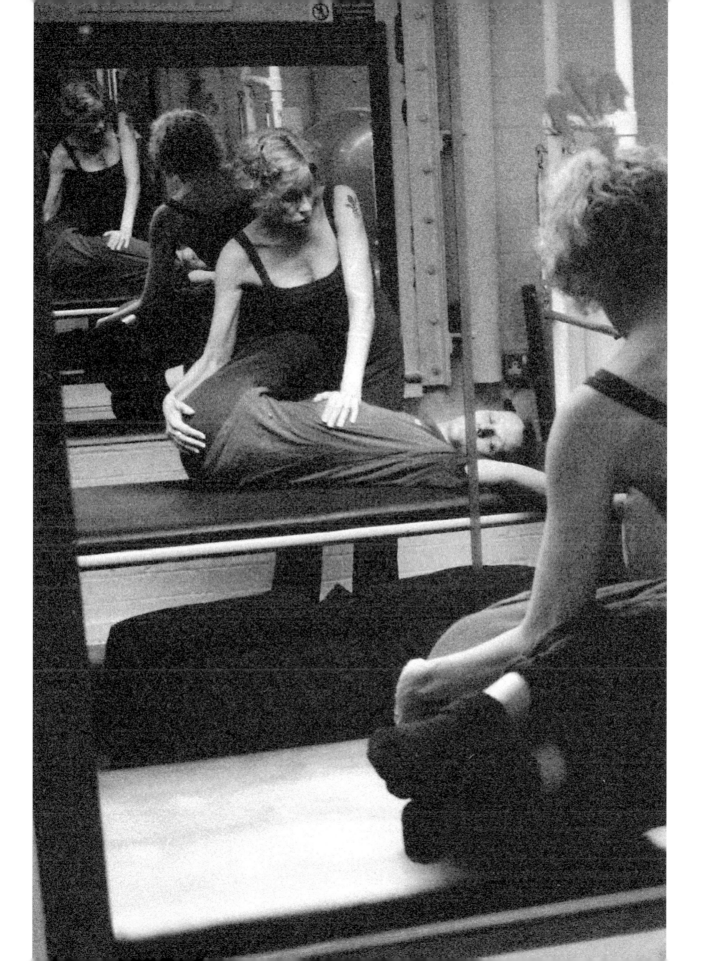

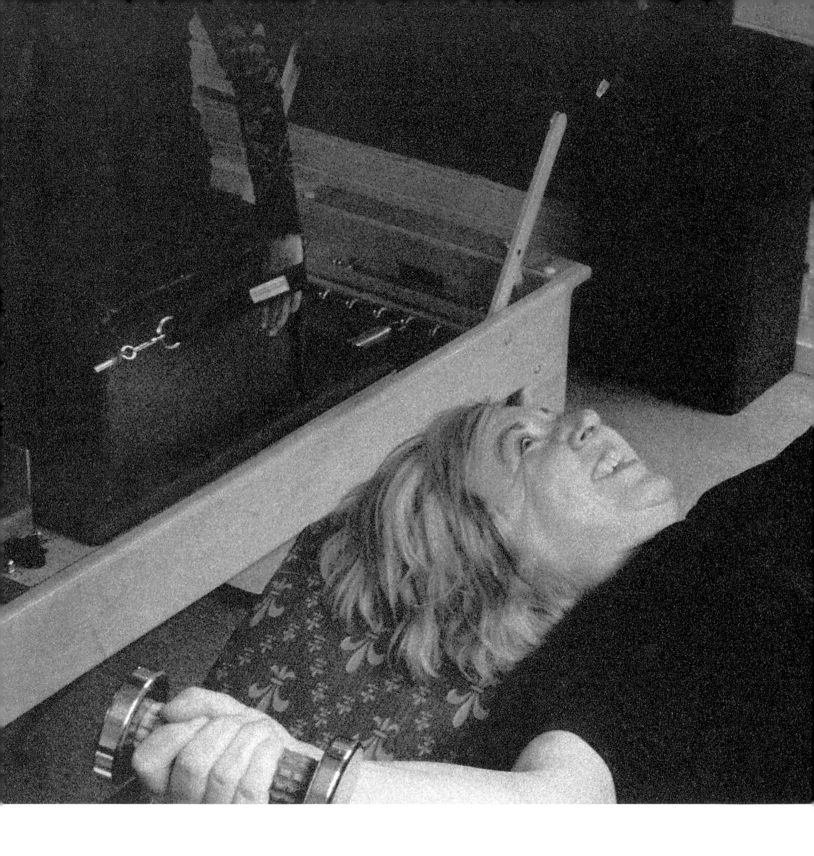

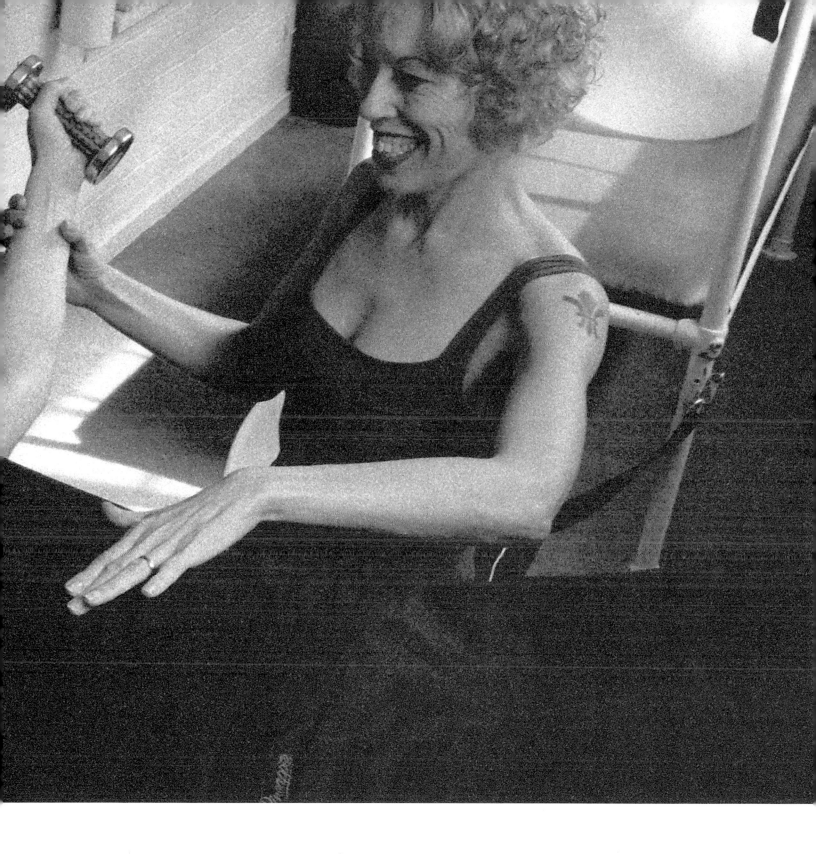

5 the exercise programme

The exercises in this section will help you to tone and strengthen specific muscles in your arms, back, stomach, chest and legs. In time, as your body adapts, you will also start to look taller, slimmer and more youthful. In addition to improving your physical shape, strength and flexibility, some of these exercises will be very helpful if you suffer from any of the following medical conditions – scoliosis, repetitive strain injury (carpal tunnel syndrome), back pain and sciatica.

Before you attempt any of the exercises in the rest of the core programme, start with the following essential posture and balance exercises. It is best to do these in bare feet. If you've got a mirror – even better. That way, if you stand sideways, you'll be able to keep an eye on what you're doing and make sure that it's correct.

PERFECT POSTURE – HOW TO LOOK INSTANTLY TALLER AND SLIMMER

Not sure if you're standing correctly? Then practise this position for a few minutes daily. After a while it will feel so natural that you no longer have to think about it.

Stand with your feet hip-width apart. Imagine that you're standing on sand. Your feet are relaxed. Think of your weight being over the middle of each foot, with your toes gently lengthening into the sand. Close your eyes and make a mental note of the following:

▷ Don't sink back into your heels or lean forward. Keep your weight evenly distributed over your feet.

▷ Let your arms fall naturally in front of your body.

▷ Let your hands hang from the shoulders, totally loose and relaxed.

▷ Don't lock your knees. They should feel relaxed and not rigid.

▷ Keep your inside thighs and bottom relaxed.

▷ Imagine that your head is like one of those nodding dogs in the back of car. It's not going backwards and forwards but resting directly upon your shoulders and rocking gently until it settles into a comfortable, neutral position.

▷ Think of the bones directly behind your ears. Try to imagine them 'reaching' towards the ceiling.

▷ Pull your stomach in, without tipping the pelvis forward. Think of a piece of string from your pubic bone to your navel. It is shortening as you pull up and in. Feel your tailbone drop – as if it is weighted to the floor. This will seem much easier after you've done more of the stretches to release the pelvic girdle.

▷ Keep the front of your thighs relaxed.

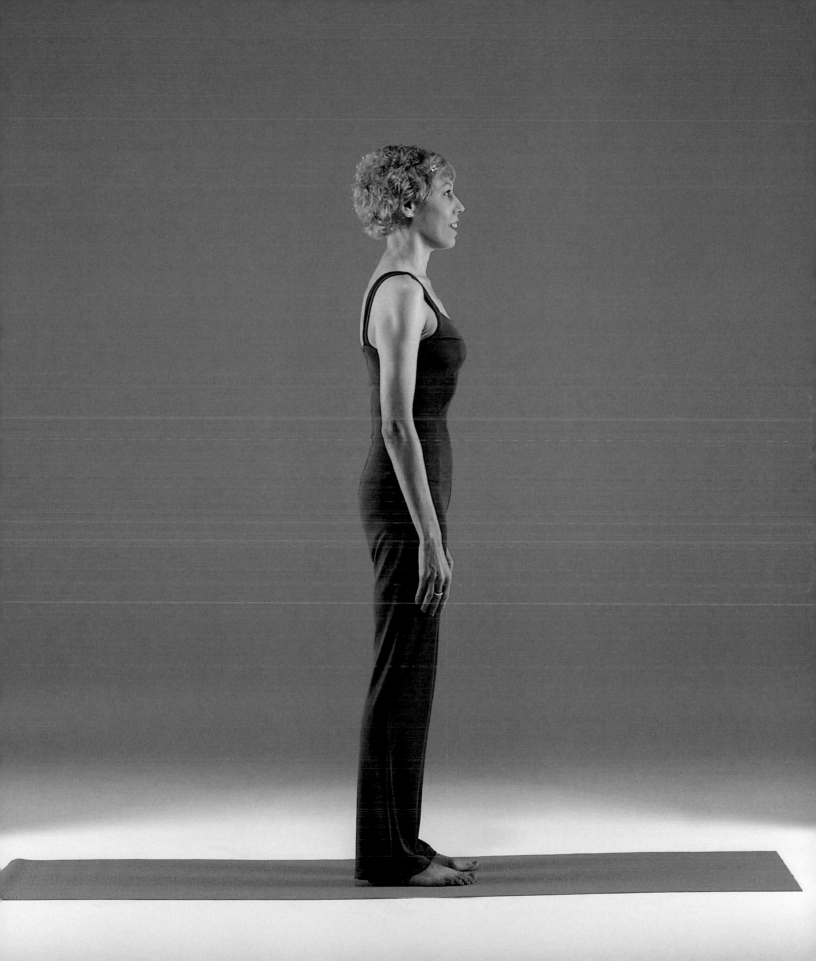

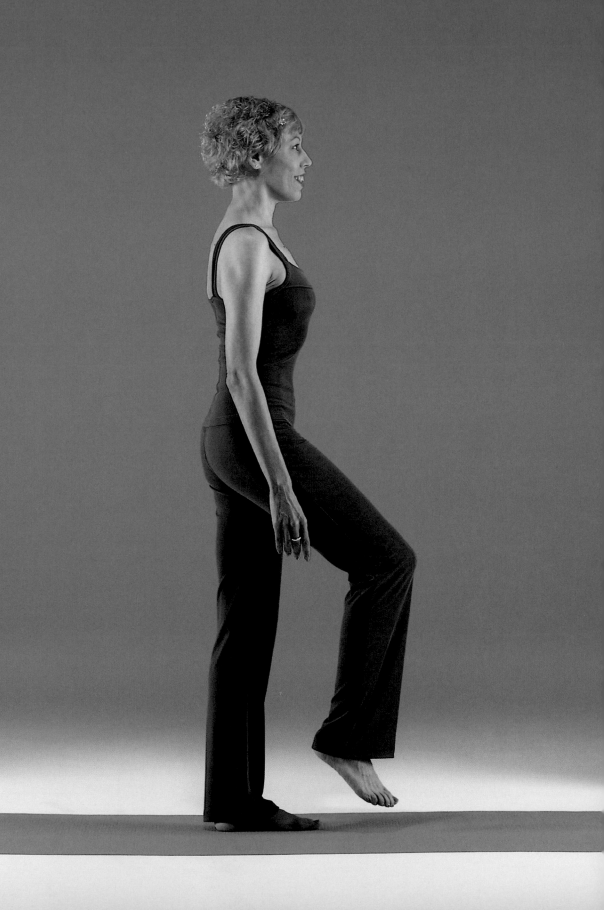

Now your whole body is perfectly aligned – you should feel as if you are floating an inch off the ground.

EXERCISES FOR BETTER BALANCE

If you're worried about slipping, tripping or not being able to catch objects thrown towards you, your sense of balance is probably poor. What seems to occur, as you get older or as a result of any injury, is that you lose your awareness of balance and your reflexes are no longer as sharp. This can cause great feelings of insecurity. Perhaps you begin to worry more about safety. We all know that the simplest of falls might have serious consequences. This is reflected in the body, which becomes stiff and constricted as a result. The easiest way to change this is to practise the following exercises every day. In time, you will start to feel lighter and more confident in the way you move.

For each of these exercises all the same rules as the 'perfect posture' exercise apply (see the checklist above).

Standing on One Leg

▷ With bare feet, stand on both legs, and imagine you are on a beach with soft sand between your toes. Let one foot float off the ground.
▷ Count for ten seconds and change legs. Repeat four times, twice on each leg.
▷ Now do the same – with your eyes closed. Make sure you have something to hold on to, lest you fall over.

Standing on One Leg on a Towel

Do exactly the same as in the previous exercise, standing on a flat towel. This gives you a slightly more unstable surface and makes the exercise more difficult. Even if you don't regularly exercise, try to do these every day – especially if you are over 45.

Walking Backwards

Start in the 'perfect posture' position and, with feet approximately an inch apart, start to walk backwards. Slowly drag your foot back, so that it never entirely leaves the floor. The easiest way to master this is to imagine that you are trying to remove some chewing gum from under your feet.

Look in the mirror – but do not look down at your feet. This exercise is even more effective if you imagine you are walking on sand.

BREATHING

Correct breathing is a very important facet of Pilates. By remembering to breathe properly, you'll find it becomes much easier to exercise. The problem is that most people don't breathe deeply enough. Breathing slowly and deeply is very energizing. It ensures there is sufficient oxygen circulating throughout the body.

It may sound obvious, but when you exercise do not hold your breath. It's better to breathe incorrectly than not at all. Practise the following exercise before you start any of the stomach work.

Basic Breathing Exercise

▷ Lie on your back in a relaxed position, resting your head on a folded towel, with your knees bent.
▷ Place one hand on your stomach and, very gently, breathe in through your nose. Feel your lungs filling with oxygen and slowly expand and relax your stomach. Breathe out.
▷ With one finger on your pubic bone and one on your navel, try and shorten that gap as you breathe out, and flatten your stomach to your spine without tilting your pelvis.
▷ Breathe in again and feel that gap slightly expand.
▷ Breathe out. Imagine there is a piece of string or an elastic band that links your pubic bone to your navel. Very gently feel it pulling up and in. This will get all three sets of stomach muscles working, including your oblique muscles, which will tighten your waist.

Make sure you breathe slowly and deeply. One of the main rules of Pilates is to breathe out on the point of effort. If in doubt, particularly on the stretches – breathe naturally.

When you breathe in your stomach gently expands. However, it shouldn't swell in an exaggerated way. Try and think of your ribcage expanding gently to the sides so that you're not just breathing into your throat and upper chest.

When you begin this exercise programme and you start to breathe properly you might feel a bit dizzy. As you are learning to breathe more deeply, you are taking in more oxygen, which can make you feel light-headed.

Abdominal and Back Exercises

Women are often obsessed with having flat stomachs like men, regardless of the obvious physical differences. These exercises, combined with careful and healthy eating, will tone and tighten the stomach area. They will not make you lose weight, but they will give you a flatter, leaner stomach.

As people age, their metabolism changes and they must exercise more to burn up the same amount of calories. By exercise, I mean walking instead of taking the car or a bus, or climbing the stairs instead of taking a lift. If you're short-waisted and eat large meals, you are going to have a stomach that protrudes. It is better for your blood sugar levels to eat small amounts throughout the day. Also allow yourself some flexibility, and don't obsessively deny yourself certain foods.

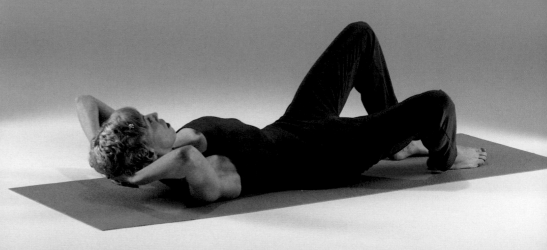

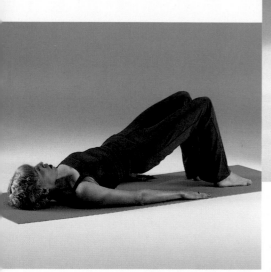

In Pilates when you do your abdominal work, as you breathe in the stomach gently expands. As you breathe out the stomach pulls in, navel to spine. Feel the connection from the pubic bone up to the navel. The body will automatically want to do the opposite as you breathe out on the point of effort. You inhale through the nose and exhale through the mouth. As you breathe out think about pulling the navel to the spine without tipping the pelvis. If you have trouble with the pelvis and you have tight hip flexors and glutes, go to the section of the leg stretches where you stretch your bottom with the foot on the thigh (see page 82), and do one or two of those stretches first to relax your pelvis.

A strong stomach exists to support your internal organs and back. The taller you stand, the more balanced your stance, the flatter your stomach will appear. When you are posturally aligned and maintaining an erect back while walking,

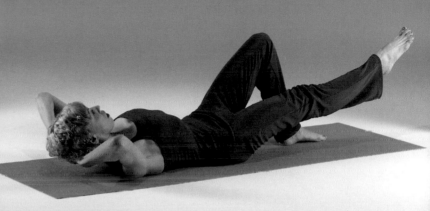

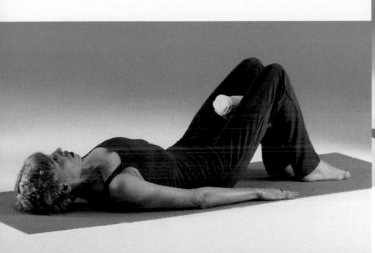

you are exercising your body perfectly well. If you sit slouched all the time and if you walk with a slump, your stomach will stick out. These abdominal and back exercises are good for conditioning, toning and strengthening. They're also good for anyone with a bad back, sciatica or scoliosis. If you have any of these problems you need to do abdominal and back work, but do not attempt any of the advanced exercises at first.

It's better to do these exercises either lying on a towel or on an exercise mat. As you're lying on your back, you may want to place a folded towel under your head. This will help lengthen your neck. If you're not sure about this, try it with and without a small folded towel and see which is more comfortable.

Repeat each exercise 10 times. Do the stretches in sets of four. Stomach muscles have an unusually short memory. Daily reminders will keep them taut and toned.

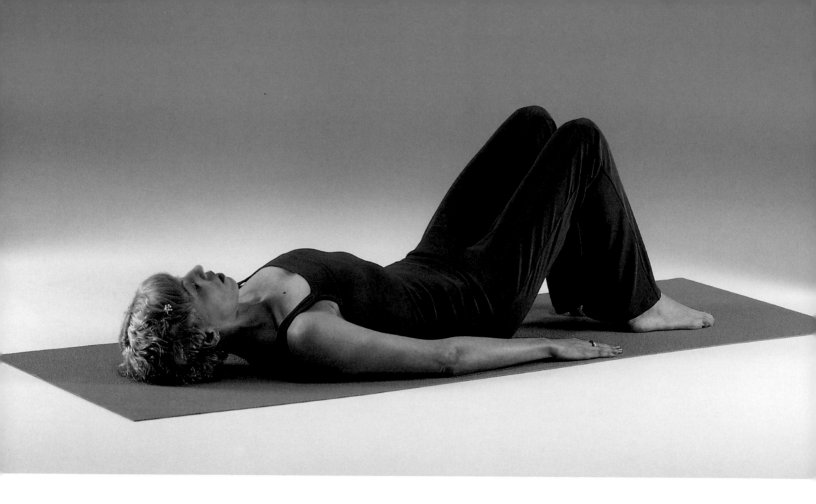

Pelvic Tilt

The pelvic tilt is a preparation exercise that warms up the back. It's a good starting point, whatever part of the programme you plan to do.

Lie on your back, with your knees bent and parallel, about hip-width apart. Arms should be resting at your sides, with palms facing the floor. This helps to lengthen your neck. Breathe in, then breathe out and gently relax your back into the floor. When you do this, do not press your back too strongly to the ground so that you lose your natural curve. Do not allow your back to arch to the point that it lifts off the floor. This is called the neutral spine position and it is slightly different for everybody (see page 19). There is no point in trying to force your back down. Try very hard not to tense your buttock muscles during this exercise.

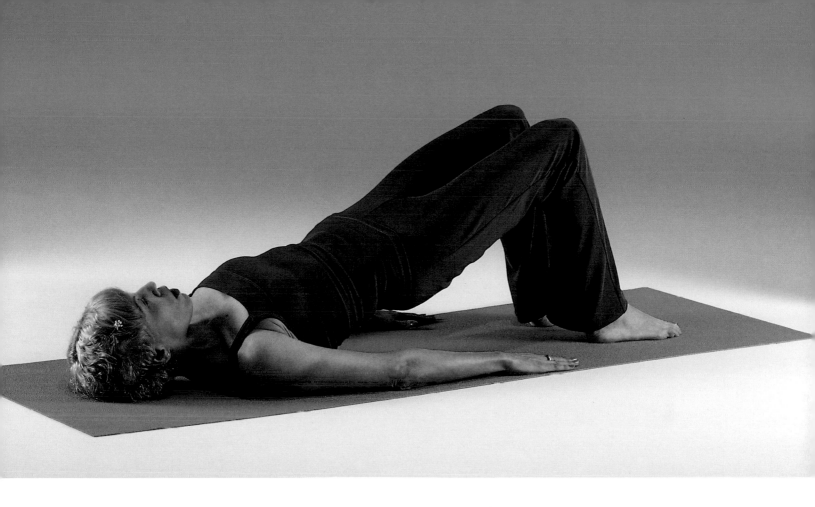

As you breathe out gently tilt your pelvis forward and roll your lower back off the floor – one vertebra at a time, as you 'peel' your back off the mat (see page 21). Breathe in, keeping your neck long, and very slowly roll all the way down, breathing out. Keep your feet relaxed on the floor and imagine that your toes are 'lengthening' away.

Preparation for abdominals

This is a preparation for the abdominal exercises. It will wake up your stomach muscles and prepare you for the more difficult exercises.

Lie as before – with a relaxed back and long neck, without tucking the pelvis under. Take either a small cushion or folded towel and place it between your thighs. Very gently breathe in through your nose. As you breathe out, feel your stomach muscles pulling down to the floor. Think of them pulling up and into your spine. Hold your breath and count to four. Squeeze the towel or cushion with your thighs. You can put your fingers on your stomach if you wish so that you can feel the muscles you are working.

As you breathe in through your nose, feel your stomach gently expand into your fingers. As you breathe out, feel your stomach pull away from your fingers. Feel your lower abdominal muscles working. Think of working on the transverse and the rectus abdominis muscles first, and the obliques second. Repeat 10 times.

WATCHPOINTS

▷ Don't let your pelvis lift off the floor. This will 'shorten' the neck. Watch that your stomach doesn't 'bloat'. Instead, make sure that on the point of relaxation – when you breathe in – the stomach gently lifts. As you breathe out you should feel your stomach pull up and in, away from the pubic bone.

▷ Most people naturally want to breathe in and pull their stomach muscles in – this is a mistake. As you breathe in, you gently soften the muscles as they flow out into your fingers. As you breathe out the stomach pulls away from the fingers. Think of it as pulling 'up and in'. This will help you focus on your lower abdominals – strengthening and toning that area.

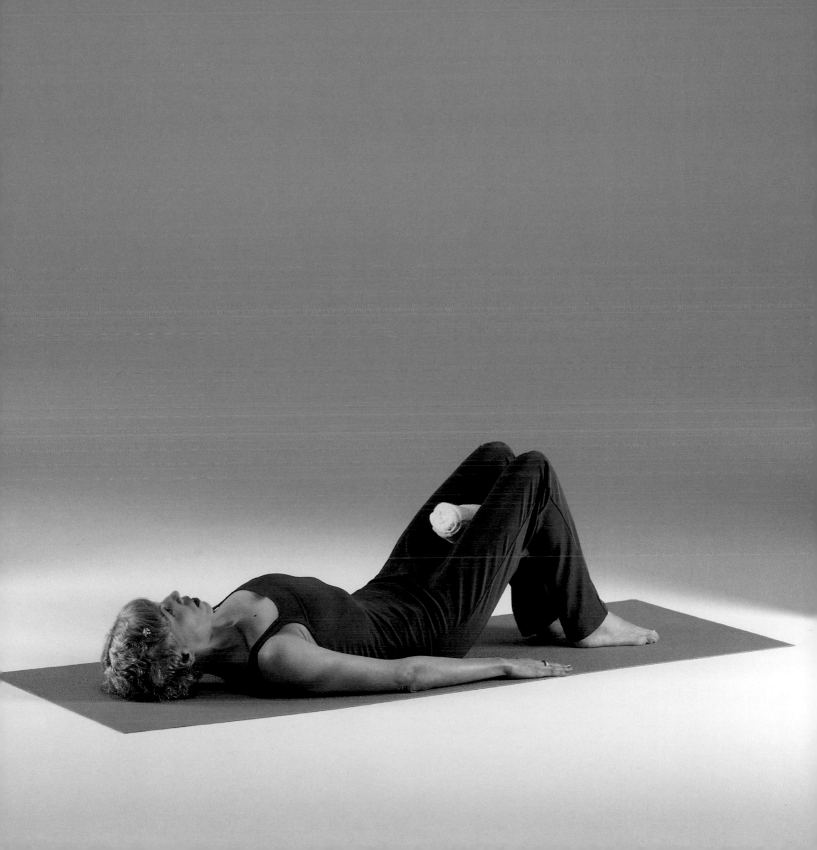

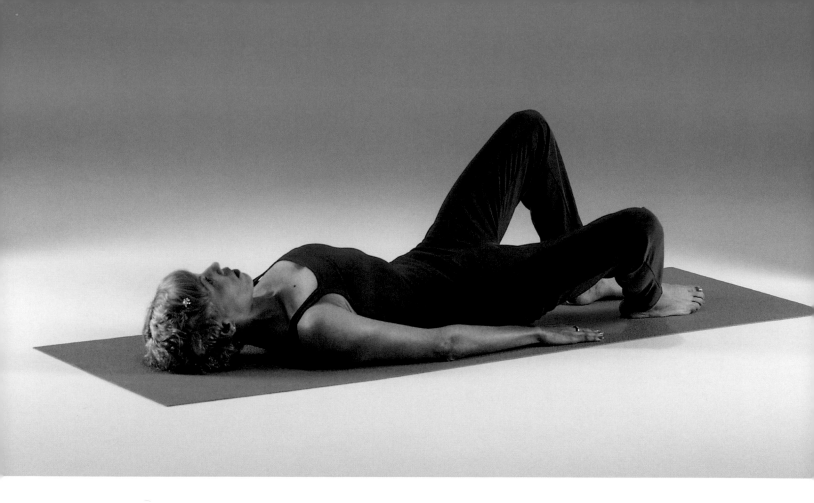

Working the Lower Abdominal Muscles

Lie in the same position as above, knees bent. You can place your hands on your hipbones. This helps to stabilize your pelvis. Begin with the right leg. Keep your left leg completely still. Very gently breathe in and let your right knee open sideways. As you breathe out feel the resistance. Bring the leg back to the other one – breathing out and pulling your stomach in. Change legs. Now, breathing in, open the left leg to the side. Exhale and slowly close. Repeat 10 times, alternating legs each time.

WATCHPOINTS

▷ Think of the muscles between your navel and your pubic bone as a fan. As you inhale and the knee opens to the side the fan opens. As you exhale, the muscles tighten and the fan closes.

▷ Don't tilt the pelvis, and make sure that the supporting side is stable.

▷ Don't press your back into the mat.

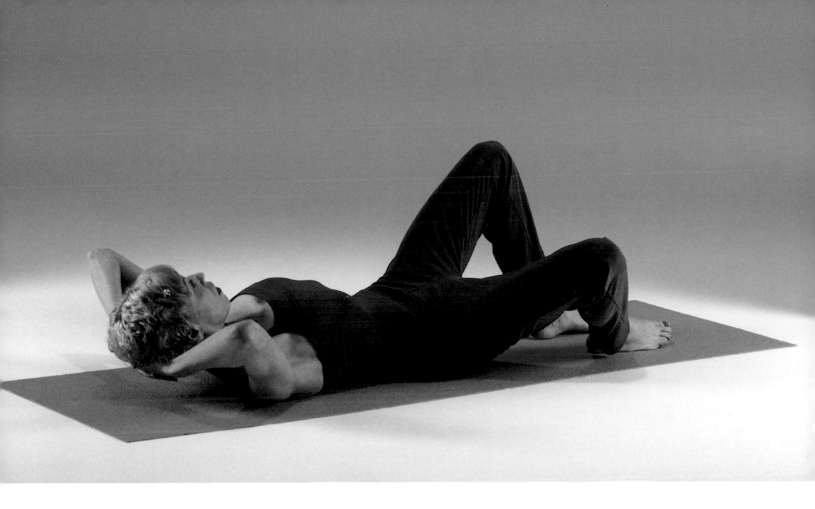

Working the Lower Abdominal Muscles 2

This slightly harder version of the previous exercise is very straightforward. Interlace your hands behind your head. (This will help prevent you from straining the muscles in your neck.) Slide them high up behind your skull. Do not let them slip to the neck. Keep thumbs on either side of your spine.

Lift your elbows so that you can just see them out of the corner of your eye without moving your head. When you can see your elbows peripherally you know that your arms are in the right place. Very gently exhale and 'float' your head and shoulders off the mat. Hold that position and repeat the previous exercise. Repeat the exercise 10 times, five times on each side.

WATCHPOINT

▷ As you lift your head, your focus shouldn't change, so you don't shorten your neck. If you shorten your neck you may tip your pelvis. This makes it very hard to work your lower abdominal muscles. You may also place a strain on your lower back and your body will be incorrectly aligned.

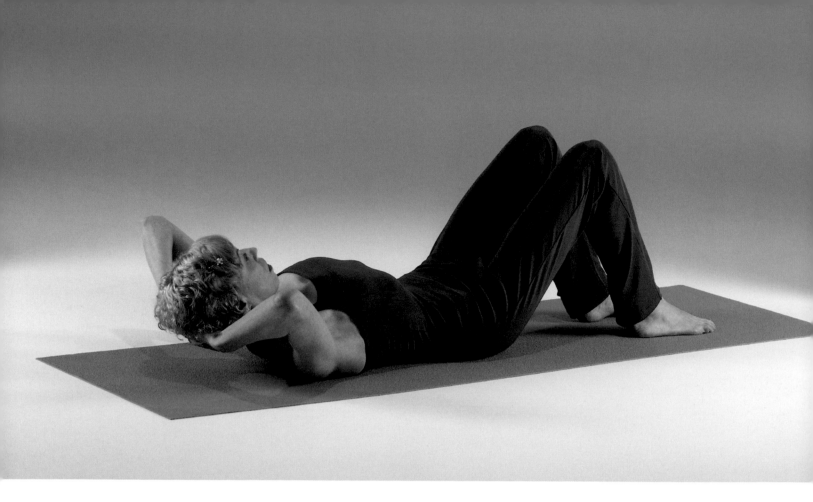

Basic Abdominal Curl

This exercise uses exactly the same position as the
previous exercise, although the knee does not fan out. All
the same rules apply. Lift your elbows up where you can
see them in peripheral vision. Keep looking at the ceiling
and gently breathe in through your nose. Relax the
abdomen, but do not 'bloat' it out. As you breathe out,
gently lift your head and shoulders off the mat. Only go
as high as you can. Do not strain your neck to hold that
position. Breathe in as you go back down again.

WATCHPOINT

▷ As you breathe out, imagine that a piece of string is
pulling you up from your pubic bone and under
your rib cage. Pause until all three sets of
abdominal muscles go 'up and in', and flatten.

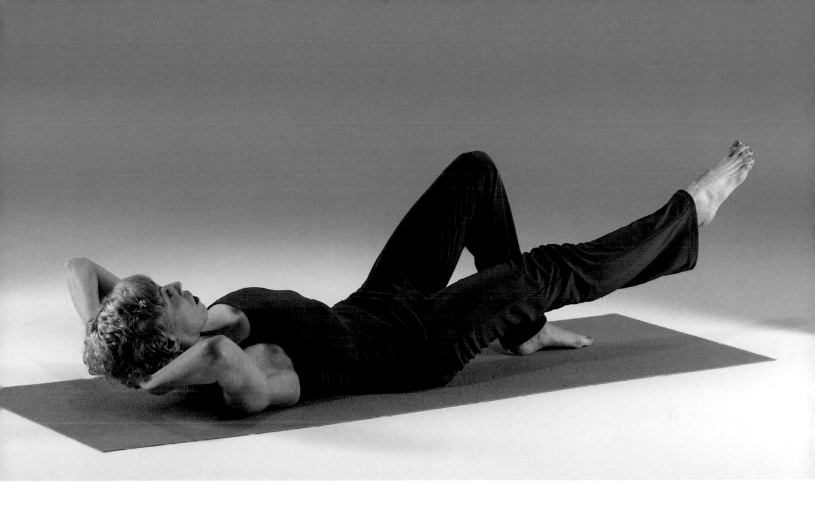

Single Leg Stretch

This stomach exercise is a simple single leg stretch. It is the first really coordinated exercise. It is a simple and basic exercise – which is not the same as saying it is easy.

Start in the same position as the exercises above and interlace your hands behind your head. Lift your head and shoulders gently off the mat. As you breathe out, slide your right leg down, an inch off the floor. Breathe in, putting your head down and bringing your right leg back up. Breathe out, and slide your left leg down, an inch off the floor. Repeat 10 times, alternating the legs.

WATCHPOINTS

▷ Many people make the mistake of exhaling before curling forward. If you do this, you will not get the same benefit. You exhale as you do the exercise.

▷ Remember to keep looking at that same point on the ceiling. If you pull your chin into your chest you may strain your neck and won't get the results you want.

Basic Sit-Up

Lie on your back with your legs comfortably against a wall or with your feet held up by a friend. Be close enough to, or far away enough from, the wall so that your tailbone is weighted to the mat. If your bottom is off the ground you're too close to the wall. Conversely, if you're too far away your legs won't feel supported.

   Take your hands behind your head and lift your elbows to where you can see them in your peripheral vision. Keep the neck long.

Very gently breathe in to prepare. As you breathe out, lift the head and shoulders off the mat, pulling your stomach towards your spine. Pause, breathe in and lower. As you breathe out and lift, the stomach pulls in, the pelvis does not lift. The neck is long, the head is cradled in the hands. You are not pulling your chin to your chest. Think of the breast bone and the head as floating off the mat. Don't think of a sharp pulling movement.

Do 10 repetitions.

WATCHPOINT

▷ Hands are interlaced high up behind the cranium and are not placed behind the neck.

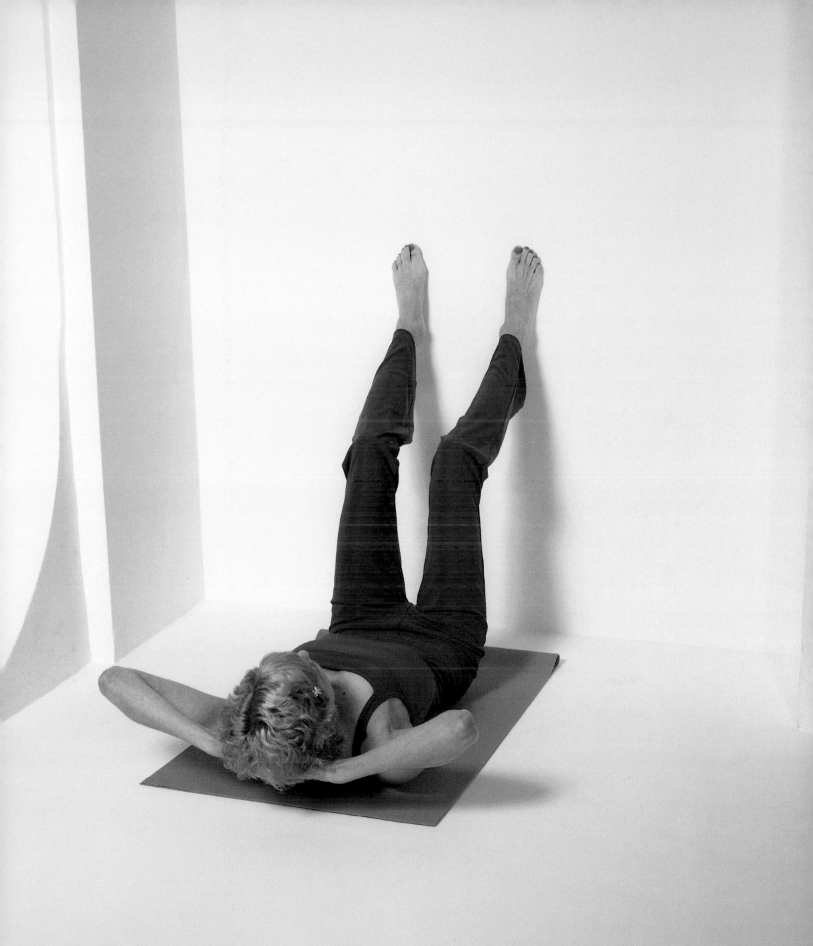

Advanced Single Leg Stretch

This is the most difficult exercise in the programme, because it is an exercise with both legs off the ground. If you have any back injuries at all, don't do it until you feel strong enough.

Bend both knees into the chest and allow your tailbone to be relaxed and heavy. Your hands are linked behind your head as before. Look at the ceiling and breathe out. Let your head and shoulders 'float' off the ground, depending on how much mobility you have. Inhale.

Exhale and stretch one leg out, pulling your stomach into the spine. Inhale and bring the leg back. Exhale and extend the other leg. Do five stretches on each leg. If you wish you may relax at the end and do another set. Only take the leg as low as the point where your back does not arch away from the floor. The lower the leg, the harder the exercise.

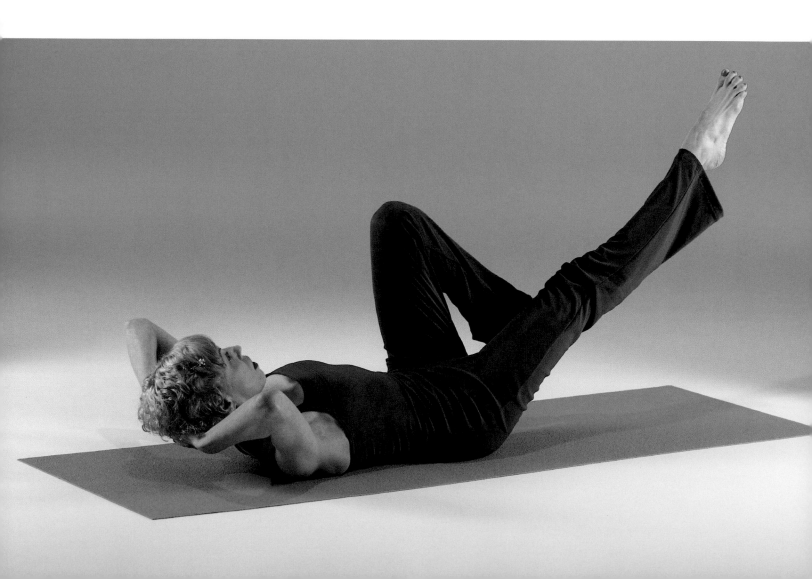

Side Stretches, Side Lifts and Back Exercises

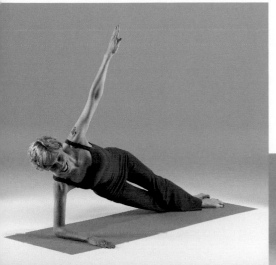

The next three exercises are also for the abdomen but they are done lying on your side. These are called side stretches and side lifts. They are particularly good for the waist obliques. The same rules apply as for all the abdominal exercises. It doesn't matter which side you lie on to start with. Do all the exercises in sets of 10. Those that follow are for the back.

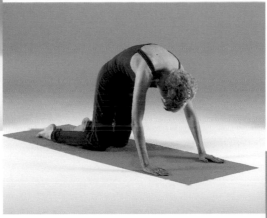

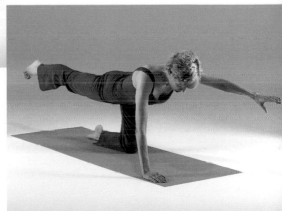

You cannot stand upright if you have a tight, weak back. Any minor adjustments that you make to try and correct the way in which you walk, sit and stand will only create further problems. Gentle exercise and control are the key. If you envision these exercises as stomach exercises, you can't go wrong. If you think of them as back exercises, the result will be frenetic movement that won't accomplish much except possibly 'concertina-ing' your bones.

If time allows, these lower back exercises should be done after the stomach exercises. These exercises work better as a pair. You must strengthen your stomach before you start working on your back, as the abdominal muscles initiate the work needed to develop a strong back. All exercises are directed from the abdominals.

Side Stretch

Lie on your side, arm stretched out in line with your body, resting on the floor, palm down. Place your other hand on the floor in front of you, for balance. If your neck doesn't feel comfortable, place a folded towel between your ear and your shoulder.

Think of your ear 'lengthening' along the arm, so that you're looking directly ahead of you. The hips are stacked one directly over the other so that your pelvis is level, not tilted. It's very common to let the top hip rock forward. Glance down your body without moving your head. If you can't see your feet, they are too far behind you. If you feel any strain in your back, the first thing you should do is move your feet further forward.

Breathe in to prepare. Breathe out and lift your legs about four inches off the ground. Keep your feet gently flexed. You want to straighten the back of your legs. Feel the energy pushing through your heels as you lift. Breathe in as you lower. Do 10 on each side.

WATCHPOINTS

▷ If you are unsure about this position, do it with your back against the wall. You can then feel how far your legs have to come forward to feel your middle back against the wall.

▷ Stretch your legs as far as you can without locking your knees. The knees are lengthened away, but slightly relaxed. If you're not sure about locking your knees or stretching your knees it's always better to have them slightly released.

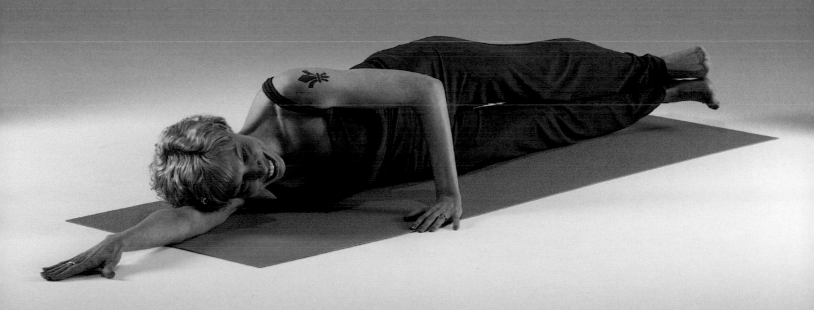

Side Stretch 2

The next exercise is simply a harder version of the one
before – so all the same rules apply. Use a towel if you
need to. Relax your top arm and shoulder. With flexed feet
breathe out and think of your legs floating off the ground.
Hold this position and breathe in. Breathe out and lift the
top leg. Bring the leg back, breathe in, and slowly lower
both legs to the ground and relax. Do 10 repetitions on
each side.

WATCHPOINTS

▷ It's really important for this exercise that you never
  allow one leg to become longer than the other. You
  don't want an imbalance in your pelvis.

▷ Correct breathing is vital. If you feel any strain in
  your back, try doing the exercise with your legs
  further forward.

Side Lift

The next exercise is more difficult and you need to be
reasonably fit to try it. Don't attempt it if you have any
back injuries.

  Lie on your side, with your elbow directly under your
shoulder, your palm flat on the floor. Keep your legs in a
straight line with your ankles crossed. It helps if can place
your feet against a hard surface – e.g., a skirting board, or
bottom of a sofa. This will give you a bit of resistance and
help you get off the ground. All the same rules on
alignment apply as in the side stretch. Keep your
shoulder and elbow in line. As you breathe out, lift,
pushing down through the supporting arm. The other
arm lifts up to a right angle in line with the shoulder.
Come back down again and relax. Begin by doing this
exercise four times on each side and slowly build up to
10. This will give you a strong, toned and, hopefully, very
trim waist.

WATCHPOINT

▷ Don't allow the top arm to swing behind you. This
  is a common fault, and can cause the body to rock
  backwards.

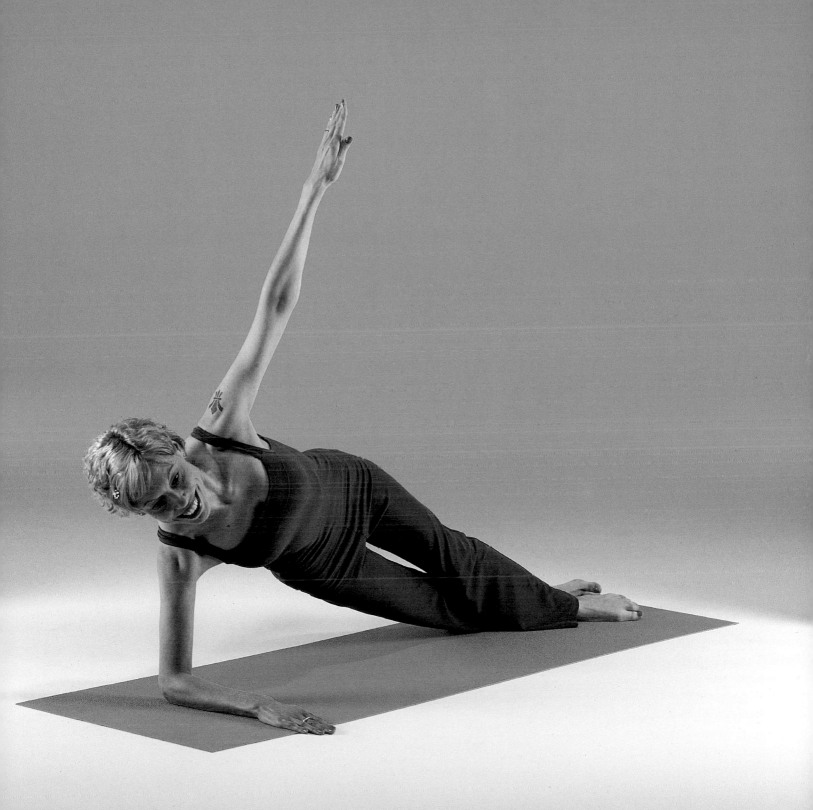

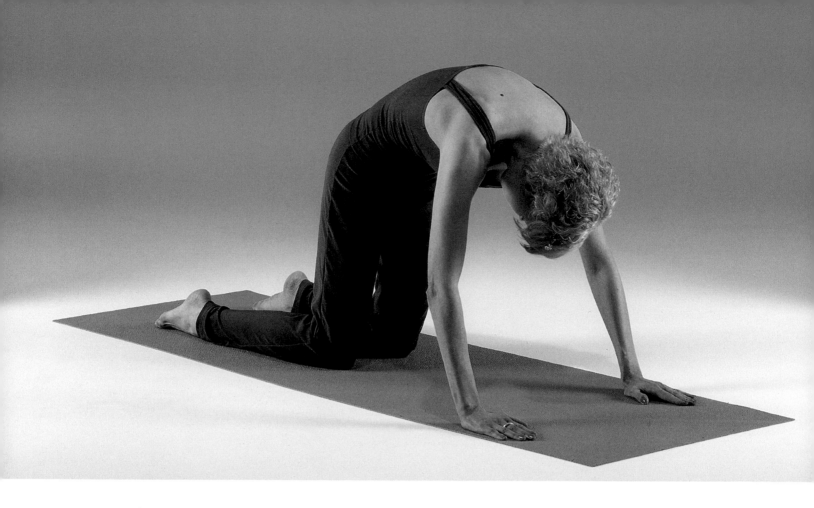

Cat Stretch

A cat stretch is done on your hands and knees. Make a square of your body. Keep your hands under your shoulders, fingers facing forwards and with your hands shoulder-width apart. Knees should be hip-width apart. If your knees feel a bit uncomfortable, just fold up a towel and put it under them. Place your feet gently on the floor and don't lock your elbows at any point. As you breathe out, drop your chin to your chest and curl your stomach into the spine. Press your upper back to the ceiling, trying not to rock back and forth. As you breathe in, your tailbone lifts towards the ceiling, your chest presses to the floor and your head gently lifts. Breathe out and reverse the position. After 10 repetitions, relax your bottom onto your heels and just breathe. This is called the 'relaxation position'. You can do this relaxation at the end of the sequence of back exercises, or at the end of each back exercise.

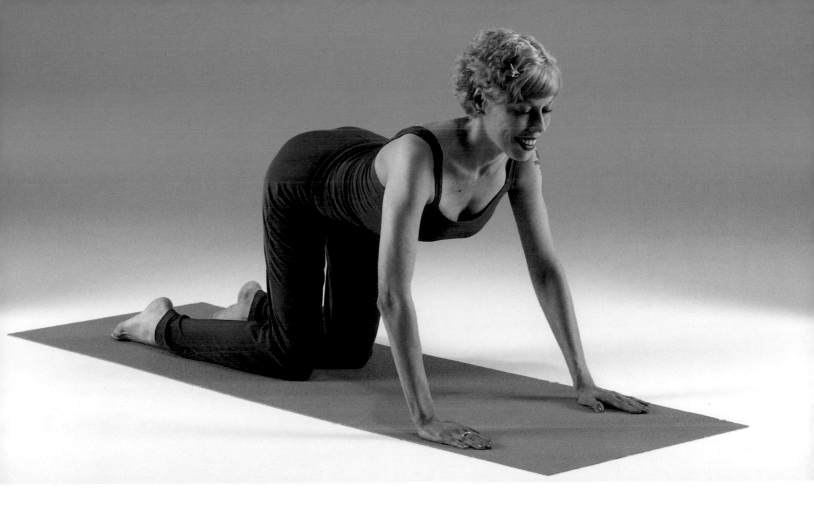

▷ Don't lock your elbows.

▷ Don't lift your head too high or you may strain your neck.

▷ As you press your chest down to the floor (in the
   reverse exercise), if you feel any pinching in your
   lower back you'll know you've gone too far.

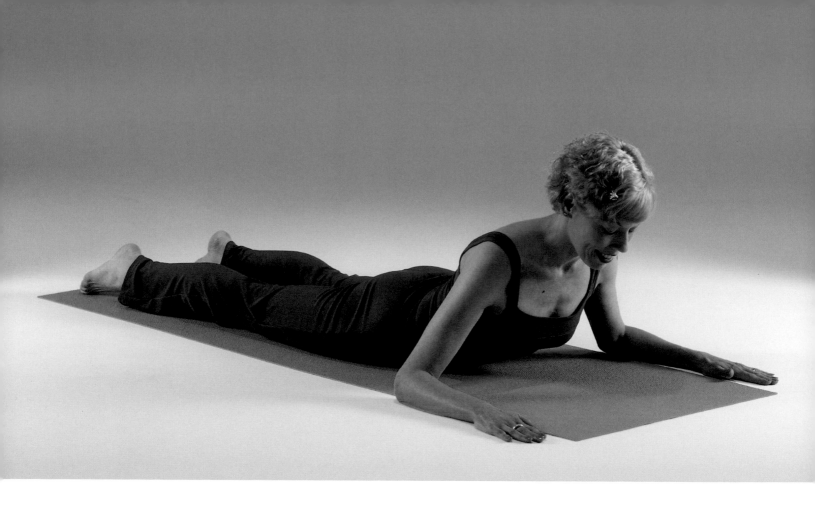

Back Strengthening

Lie on your stomach with your feet relaxed. Your arms should be facing forwards and be just wider than your shoulders, which are relaxed. Keep your neck 'long' by looking down. Keep looking down as you gently press your hips and elbows into the floor and pull your stomach in. Gently, lift your head up (keep it independent of the body), focusing your eyes on the same point. Make sure you keep your feet on the floor. Breathe in, and gently come down. Feel your buttocks contract slightly. Do not contract them too much – otherwise you're using your buttock muscles and not the stomach. Engaging the abdominals helps to strengthen your back and lift your body.

As you breathe out and lift, imagine that the crown of your head is going forward towards the wall in front of you. Do not lift your head towards the ceiling. Ideally, you want as little pressure on the hands as possible. Relax your fingers and feel your shoulder blades releasing. Relax down again.

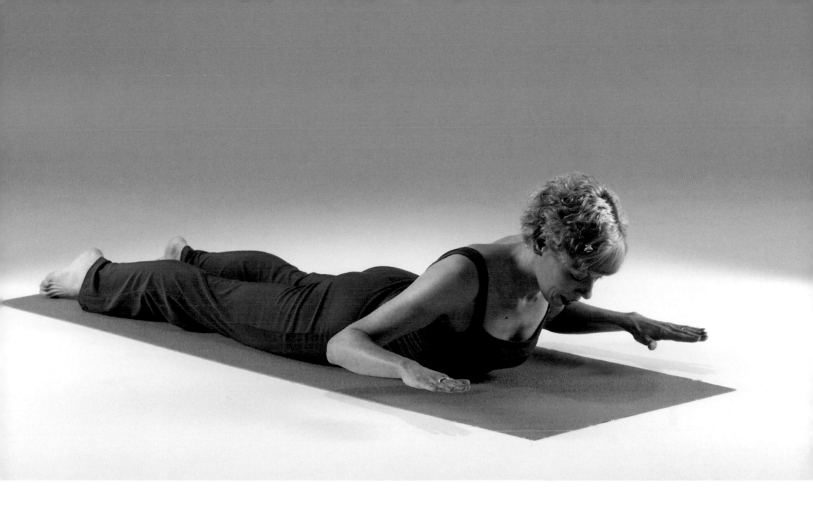

Back Strengthening 2

This exercise is exactly the same as above, except that this time, as you breathe out and lift, your hands 'float' off the ground.

▷ As you breathe out and lift, you should be able to get your fingers between your stomach and the floor.

▷ Whenever you do a back exercise, each time you breathe out, your stomach goes into the spine (just as in the earlier abdominal exercises). If you lift too high and you feel your back shortening, you've gone too far.

Alternate Arm and Leg Stretch for the Back

This works your stomach and your back.

Lying on your stomach, imagine yourself in the shape of a rather small starfish. Your arms are slightly wider than your shoulders. Look down at the floor. Make sure your legs are comfortably apart and rotated slightly outwards. Don't force it though, simply lie there and just let your legs relax into their natural position. Exhale and let your left leg and right arm gently float off the ground. Feel your stomach doing all the work. Breathe in and lower. Exhale as you change sides. Make sure that as your stomach goes in your tailbone drops. As you breathe, don't grip your bottom. Again, keep your legs straight and shoulders relaxed. Your arms and legs should be at the same height. Repeat 10 times, alternating between sides.

WATCHPOINT

▷ Don't shorten your neck, grip your bottom, or lift your arm and leg too high. Don't think of 'lifting' – you should be 'lengthening' your arm and leg. The idea here is to do a diagonal stretch that strengthens and mobilizes the big back muscle between the base of one shoulder blade and the top of the opposite buttock.

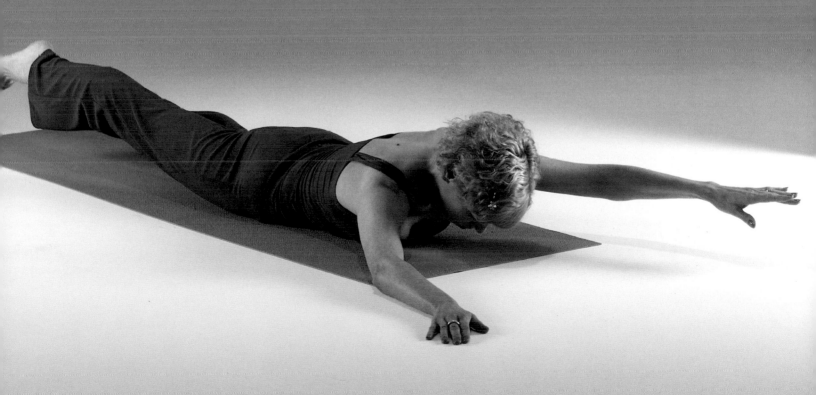

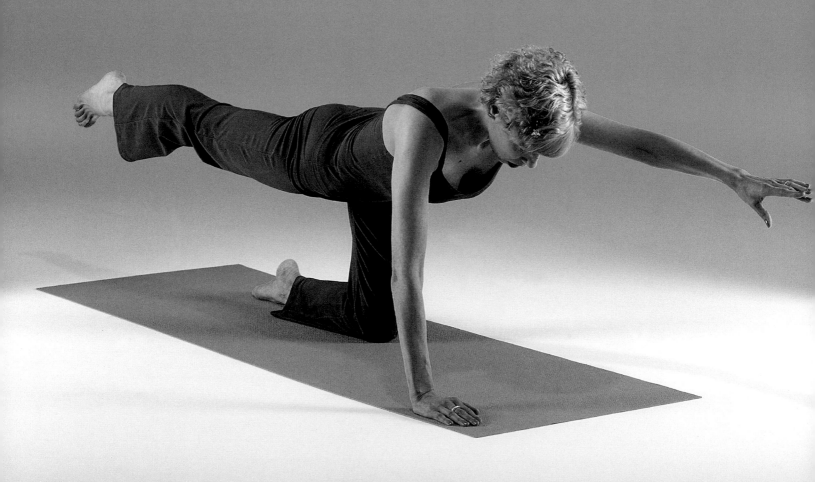

Kneeling Arm and Leg Stretch

This exercise helps improve balance.

Assume the same position as the cat stretch (see page 60). The spine is neutral and stomach gently in. Imagine someone's hand on your stomach. Breathe out, and let your right arm and left leg gently float away. Don't lift too high. To avoid this, position something like a kitchen roll across the base of your spine. If you lift too high, it will fall off. Keep your pelvis neutral, so that you don't tilt from side to side. Keep looking at the same point on the floor, so that you don't shorten your neck. Relax back into the starting position. Repeat, alternating arms and legs for 10 repetitions.

WATCHPOINT

▷ If this exercise feels too difficult at the onset, you can start by lifting one arm, or one leg only.

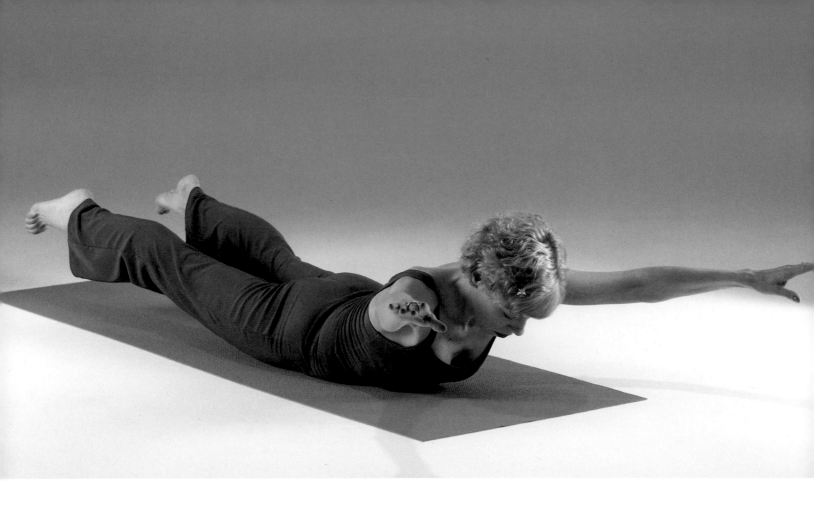

The Swan – Advanced Back Exercise

All the same rules apply as in the alternate arm and leg stretch (see page 64). Once again, imagine you are a small starfish, lying on your front, with your arms and legs comfortably apart. As you breathe out, simultaneously lift both arms and both legs to the same height. Keep looking down throughout, and pull your stomach into your spine until you feel your tailbone drop.

WATCHPOINTS

▷ Make sure that as your stomach goes in, your pelvis relaxes back; as you breathe, don't grip your bottom.

▷ Again, keep your legs straight. If you bend your knees the exercise won't be effective.

▷ Keep shoulders relaxed, stomach in, legs and arms straight. Your arms and legs should be at the same height.

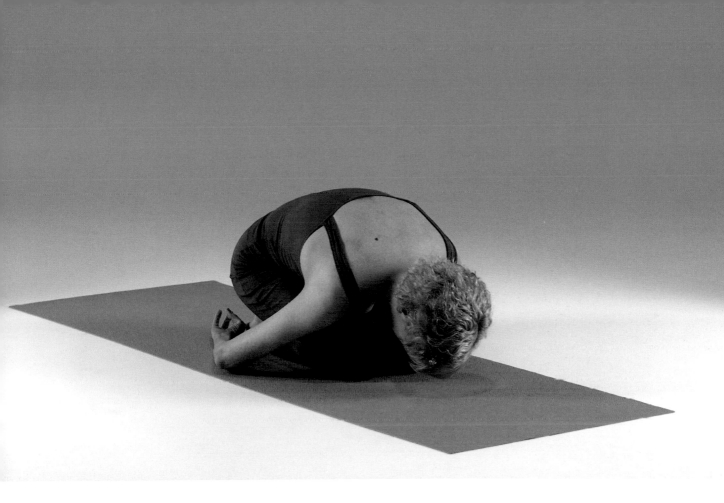

Relaxation Position – Child's Pose

Do this at the end of the back exercise sequence.

Sit back down on your heels with your arms close to your sides. Gently pull your head into your chest and curl yourself into a small 'ball' until your forehead touches the ground. Hold for a few seconds.

Legs

It is possible to create bulk by exercising the legs if you do not do enough stretching. Everyone wants their leg muscles to be long, lean and lengthened as opposed to tight and bunched. There are certain parts of the legs, particularly the quadriceps muscles above the knees, that get bigger due to excessive use, while the inside thighs and the hamstrings are usually undertoned. Many people tend to have over-developed quads, weak inside thighs and tight, but not strong, hamstrings.

The following exercises will help to strengthen, tone and condition your legs and help to make them more shapely.

Any of the following exercises can be done with ankle weights. However, don't use anything heavier than one kilo. You want to tone and lengthen muscles, not build them up.

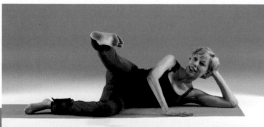

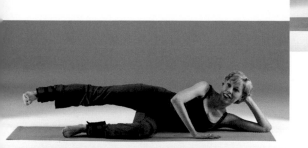

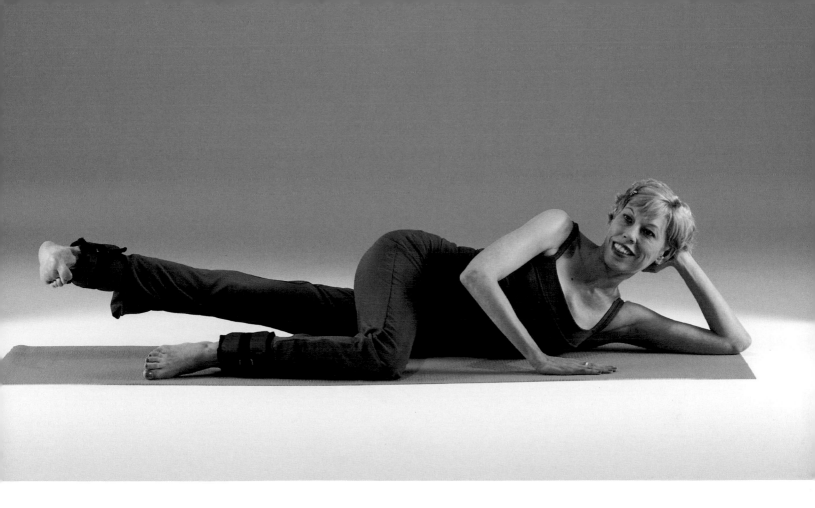

Inside Thigh Lift

This exercise will help tone flabby inside thighs.

You can do this lying on your side, either with your hand supporting your head, or with your arm completely flat. If you choose to keep your arm flat, it may feel more comfortable to put a towel between your arm and ear. Your top leg should be forward, in front of the body. If this feels awkward, place a pillow under your knee. The other hand is in front of you. The underneath leg (the one that is working) needs to be slightly forward, with your foot gently flexed. Again, don't lock your knee, but pull up the muscles, so that your leg is straight. If your legs are not straight, you'll be working your ankle and your foot much more than your inside thigh.

Breathe out, lift your leg and hold. Then slowly lower it. Don't lift your leg too high. Think of your leg going 'away',

not up – as you want to lengthen and strengthen your muscles, not have them contracted and tight. As you lift and breathe out, your stomach pulls in, just like in the earlier stomach exercises. The energy is through the heel, working your inside thigh. Do 10 on each side.

WATCHPOINT

▷ It's important to remember that, in all the leg exercises, the instigator is your stomach. This means you should feel your abdominal muscles working. The same applies to all the upper body exercises.

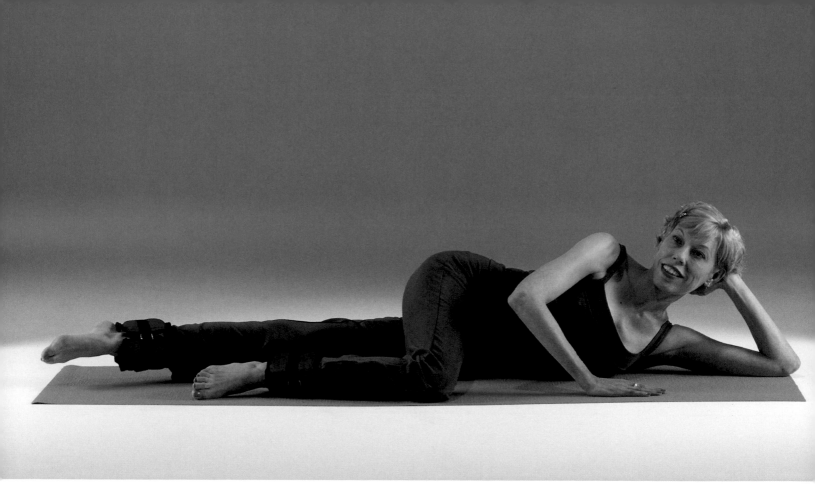

Inside Thigh Circles

Assume the same position as in the previous exercise. Gently point your foot. Breathe out and lift your leg. Slowly circle the leg in each direction. As you circle the leg, don't think of going up and down. Think of going out and away, so that you're almost touching the floor, as if you're circling around a fifty pence piece.

Do 10 little circles each way on each leg.

WATCHPOINT

▷ The knee is gently pulled up, the leg is reaching away, and you're circling down and away, not up.

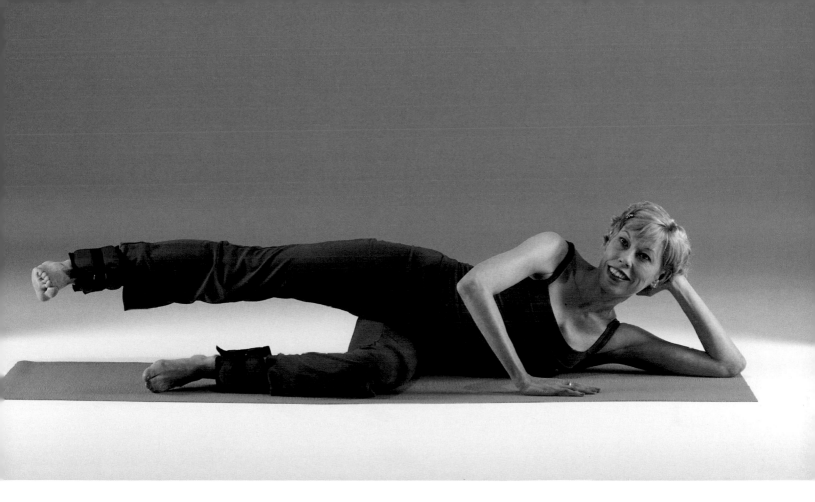

Outer Thigh Lift

To work the outer thighs and buttocks.

Take up the same position as before, only this time
your underneath leg is bent comfortably in front of you.
The top leg is straight, flexed and very slightly forward. If
you've got any doubts about your back arching, you can
lean against a wall.

The top leg should start the exercise at hip height. Very
gently breathe out and lift the leg about six inches. Don't
turn your toes towards the ceiling. Keep your foot facing
forward, gently flexed. When you breathe out and lift,
focus on the outer thigh and the back of the leg.

Do 10 on each side.

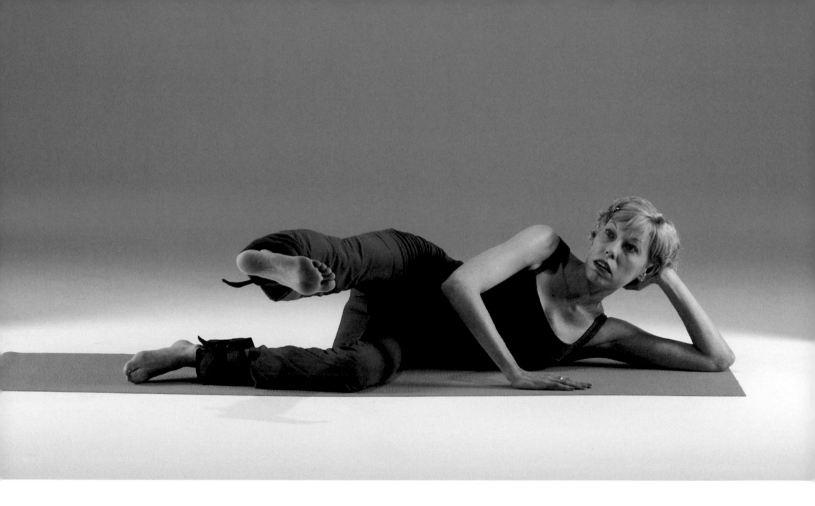

Outer Thighs and Buttocks

Start this exercise in the same position as the outer thigh lift. Make sure your top heel is in line with your hip. Very gently breathe out and bring your leg forward, so that it's in line with the other knee. Breathe in, and lift. Breathe out, and lower and take leg back. This is quite a demanding exercise, so start with five on each side, then gradually build up to 10.

WATCHPOINTS

▷ As you breathe out, and pull your leg forward, don't swing it. Think of your leg as a 'resistance', so that it is the stomach that is bringing your leg forward, up, down and back, as you tone the back of the thigh. Keep it in line with the other knee. Your hip stays back, your stomach stays in.

▷ If you find you get cramp in your hip, this exercise might not be for you.

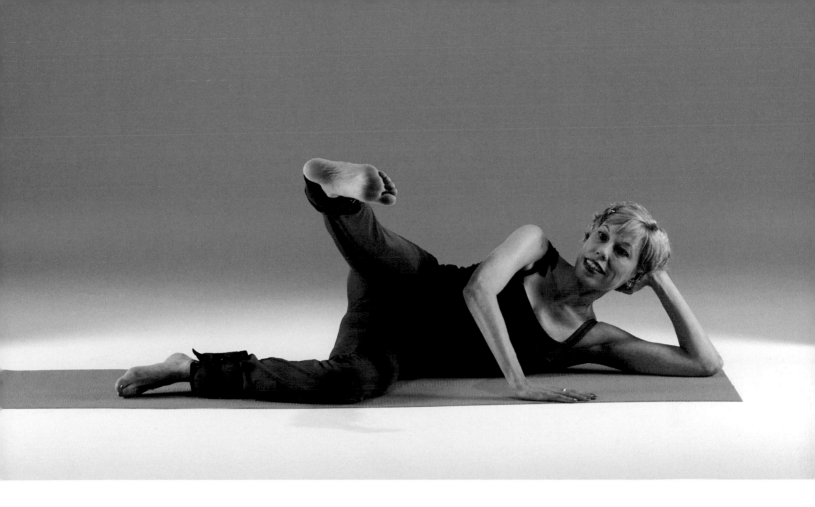

Outer Thighs and Buttocks 2

In the same position as the previous exercise, bend both
knees, so that they are comfortably in front of you. Gently
flex your feet. Lift the top leg, as if you're opening a fan.
Then very gently breathe out, and squeeze the top leg to
straight. As you breathe in, make a small bend in the
knee. Breathe out and squeeze to straight. Remember –
the emphasis is not on the bend, but on the squeeze. If
you do a big bend, you'll be working your calves, not your
bottom. Do 10 on each side.

WATCHPOINT

▷ If you get cramp, this indicates that your muscles
  are fatigued and it is best to stop.

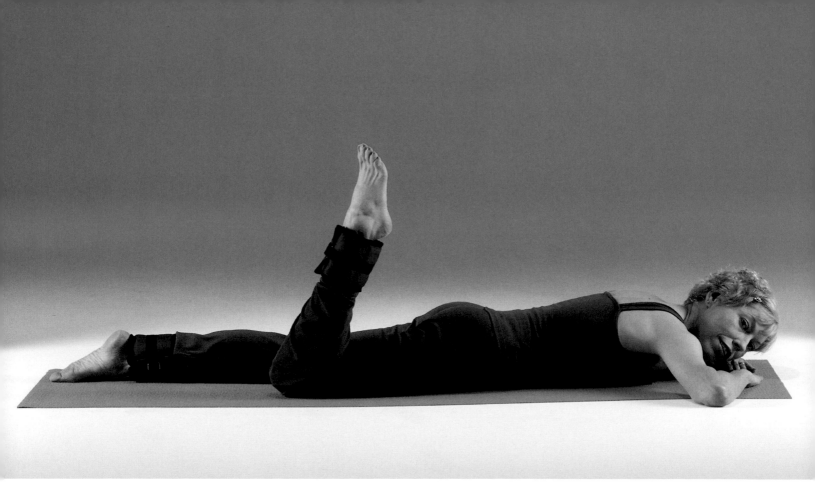

The following leg exercises are all done lying on the stomach. They can all be done with one-kilo ankle weights.

Hamstring Toner and Strengthener

Lying on your stomach, your head should be comfortably relaxed on your hands. If you prefer, keep your arms at your sides. Do whichever feels more comfortable. Keep your shoulders relaxed. Very gently 'grip' your bottom. As you do so, you should feel your stomach going in and your tailbone drop. Inhaling, bend your right leg and flex your foot. Then gently exhale and straighten, keeping the buttocks squeezed at all times. Repeat 10 times then change legs. (The bend on this exercise is not important, it's just a preparation.)

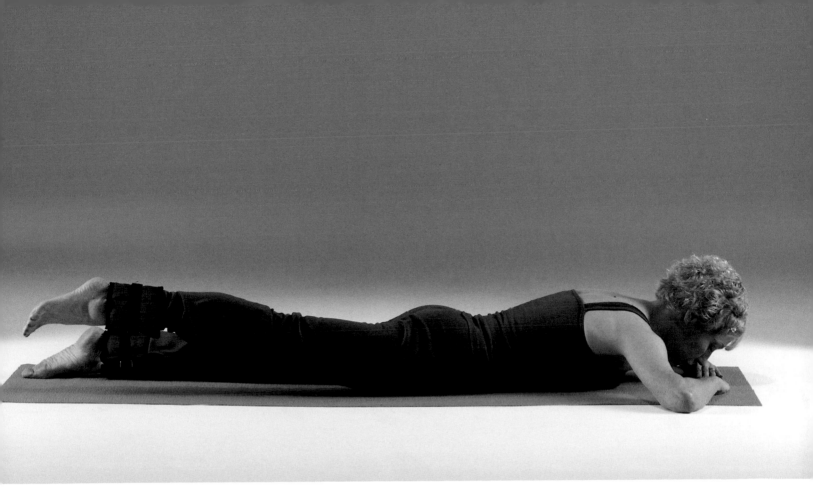

The next two exercises are similar, except for the position of the foot.

Bottom Toner

Assume the same position on your stomach as above. With a straight leg, hip down, stomach in, keeping foot relaxed, very gently breathe out and lift your leg up. Then slowly bring it down. This works the buttock muscles which are just under the cheek. Do 10 repetitions on each leg.

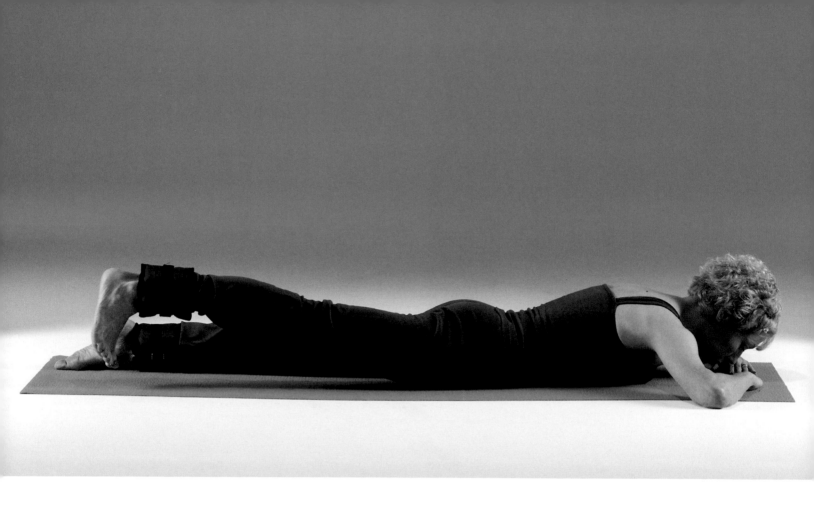

Bottom Toner 2

This is exactly the same as above, except this time as you breathe out and lift, keep your foot softly flexed. Repeat 10 times on one leg and then the other.

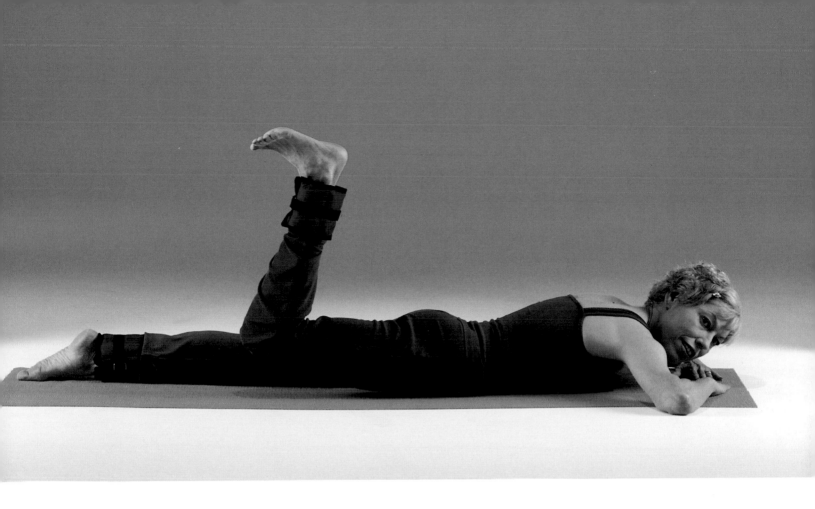

Bottom Toner 3

This is the last exercise in this sequence, and all the same rules apply as above. Starting in the same position, this time you bend your leg and flex your foot as you lift. Keep your hip down, and foot, knee and ankle in line, as you breathe out and slowly squeeze towards the ceiling.

Repeat 10 times on one leg and then the other.

▷ At no point in any of these three exercises should your hip-bones leave the mat.

▷ If you feel your back arch, place a rolled towel beneath your stomach.

Leg Stretches

It is vital that you do leg stretches after you've done any leg strengthening work. They are especially important if you have any back problems. If you've got a tight back, you may have tight legs. Sometimes it's difficult to know which comes first – a bad back and tight hamstrings, or tight hamstrings resulting in a bad back. Also, if you do have back problems you are likely to have a pelvic imbalance, which is often caused by over-tight gluteal muscles, hip flexors and quadriceps, so that your pelvis is not in line. If you can get your body in line, you'll feel much more comfortable, and you will avoid a lot of problems.

Hold all stretches for 30 seconds.

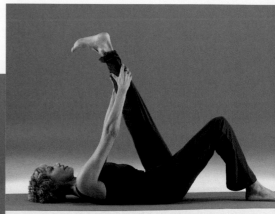

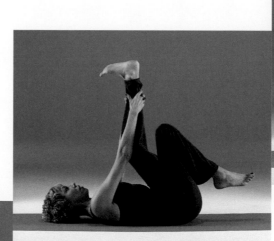

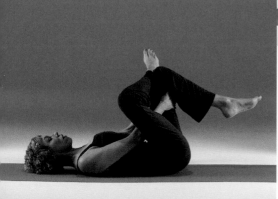

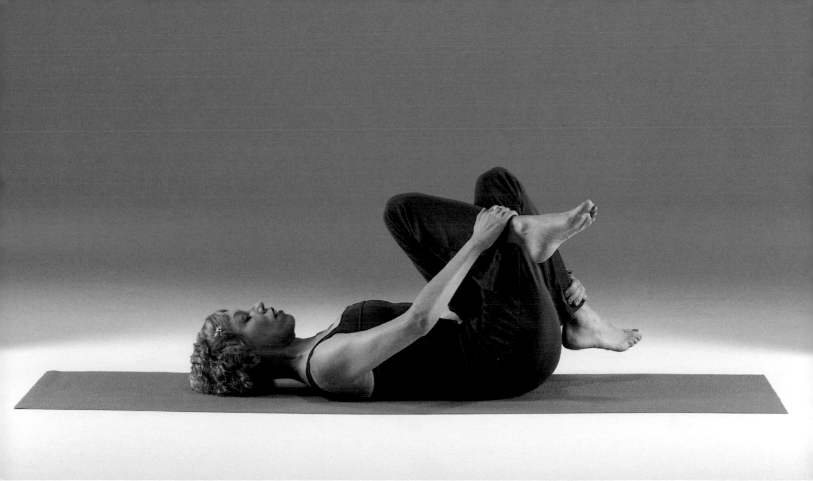

Back and Hip – Gluteal Stretch

Lying down on your back, cross your knees, hold onto
your ankles, and very gently pull your heels into your
bottom. Do this for 30 seconds with the right leg on top,
then 30 seconds with the left leg on top. Repeat four
times in total.

WATCHPOINTS

▷ Don't let your bottom lift – it should stay 'weighted'
to the ground.

▷ Don't hold onto your feet – hold onto your ankles.

▷ If it feels more comfortable, place a towel under
your head.

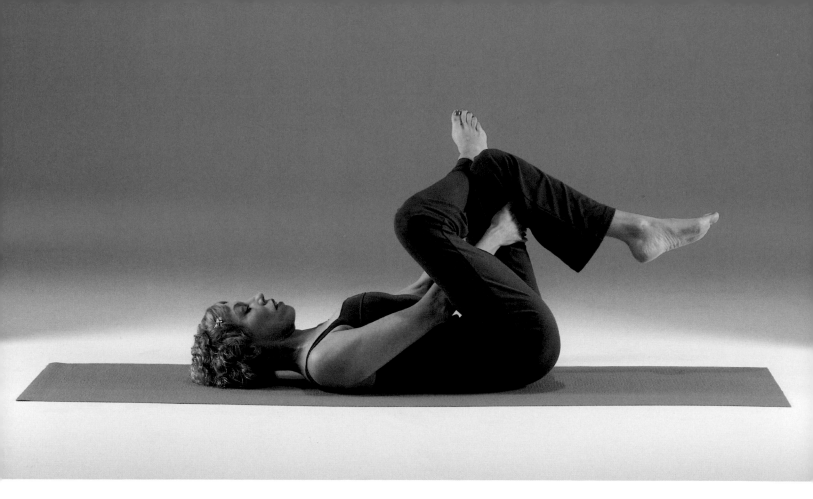

Back and Hip – Gluteal Stretch 2

This is a slightly more advanced version of the above
exercise. It will help to release the hips.
Lying on your back with your legs bent, very gently cross
the right ankle over the left knee. Make sure it's the ankle,
and not the toes. Gently, keeping your knee open, bend
the leg into the chest and feel a stretch on the bent leg.
Remember, on all the stretches, you should only feel a
stretch on the working leg. Hold for 30 seconds, change
legs and repeat four times.

WATCHPOINT

▷ With both the above exercises, if you feel a strain in
your back – stop. This means you're working your
legs too hard.

The following exercises will stretch the quadricep muscles at front of your thighs. Hold all stretches for 30 seconds.

Quadriceps Stretch

Stand upright. Hold onto something if you feel you're losing your balance. Grasp one ankle and gently stretch the front of your thigh. Keep your knees in line (check in a mirror if you're not certain). Ensure that your stomach is in, and your tailbone dropped. You should be stretching from the hip flexor all the way down to the front of your thigh. Do not arch your back. Repeat four times, alternating legs.

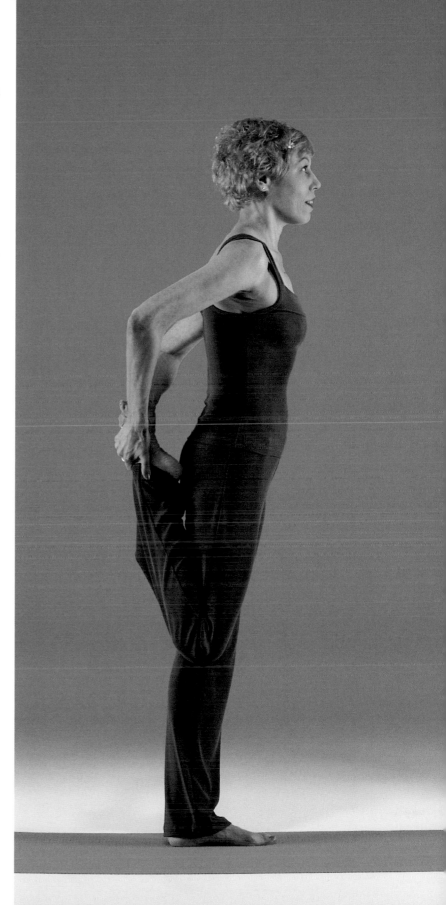

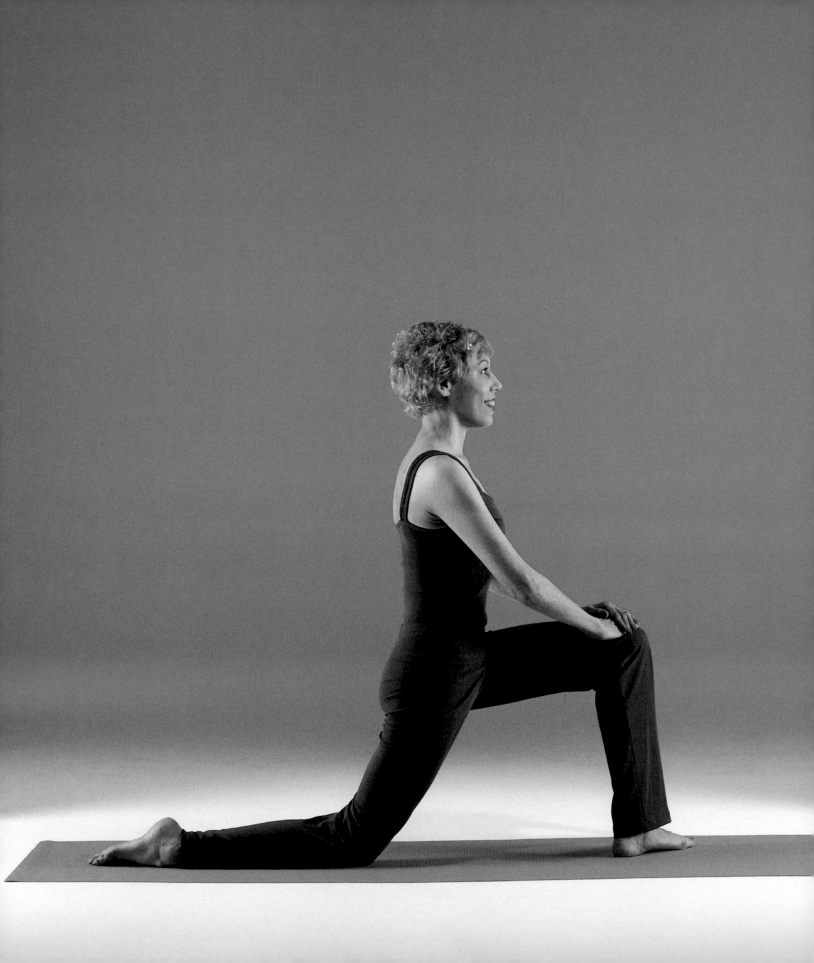

Quadriceps Stretch (advanced)

Kneel down on your right leg. Extend the left leg so that
the knee is directly over the ankle. Gently pull your
stomach in. Lean back slightly without arching your back.
Hold for 30 seconds. Repeat four times, alternating legs.

WATCHPOINT

▷ If this stretch causes pain in your knee or your back
– stop.

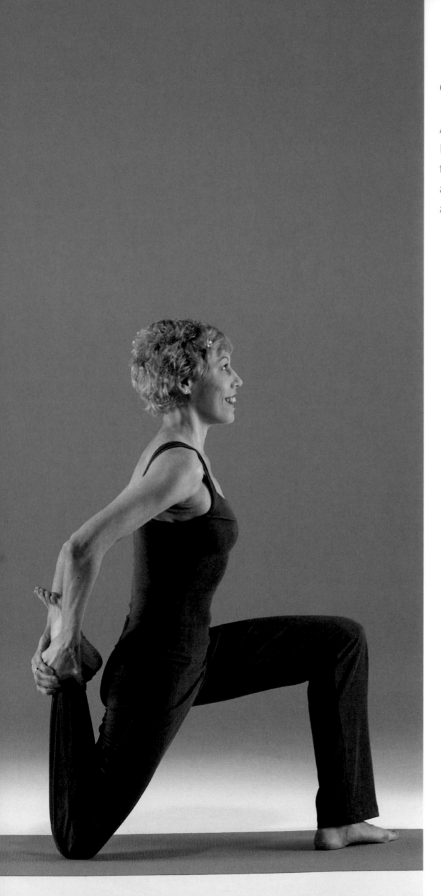

Quadriceps Stretch (advanced) 2

Assume the same position as the exercise above.
Holding your back foot, bend your knee and pull the foot
towards your bottom. Keep your stomach in and don't
arch your back. Hold for 30 seconds. Repeat four times,
alternating legs.

Lying Calf Stretch

Lying on your back, bend your knees into your chest.
Place your hand behind the calf of the leg that you're
working, and stretch the leg towards the ceiling. Keep
your foot flexed. Hold for 30 seconds. Repeat four
times, alternating legs.

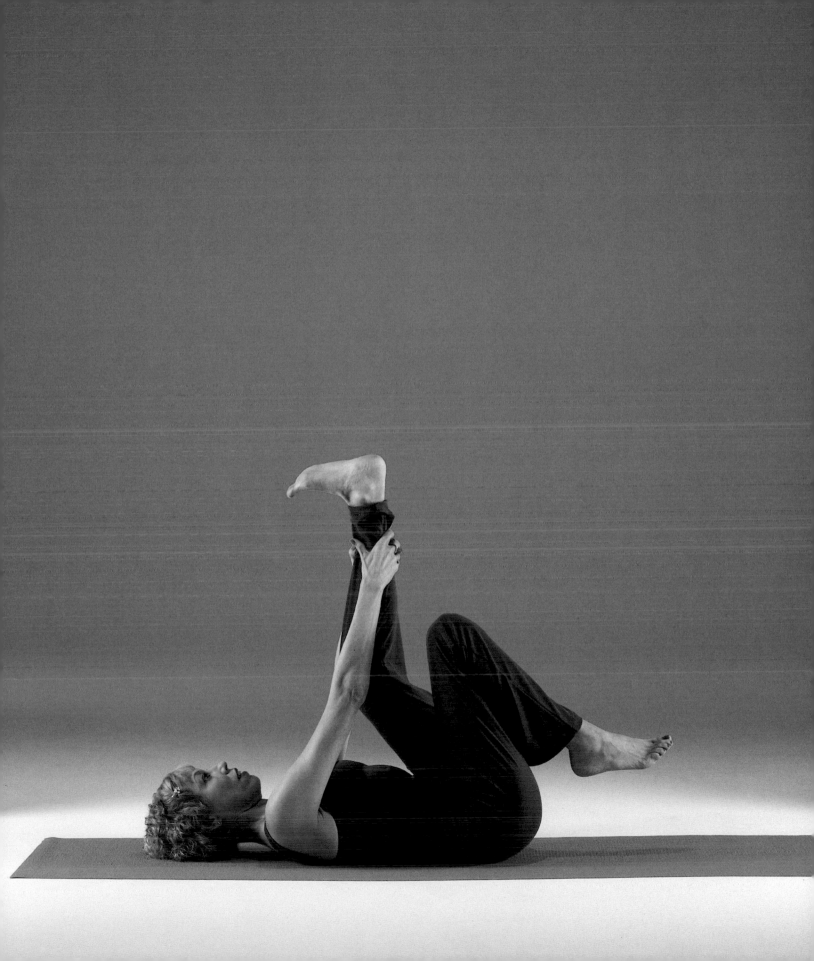

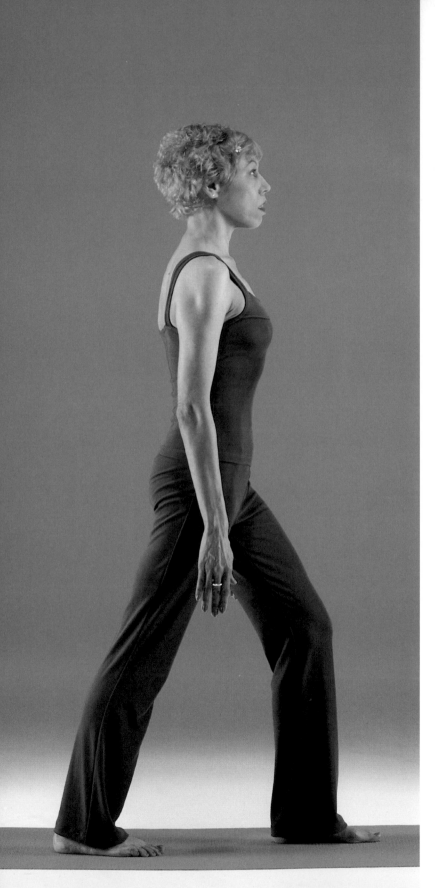

Standing Calf Stretch

Stand up straight. Take a step forward with your left leg, bend the knee slightly, and feel the stretch down through the back leg. Keep your heel down on the back leg. Do not bounce. Hold for 30 seconds. Repeat four times, alternating legs.

Standing Hamstring Stretch

Place your foot (gently flexed) on a chair and extend your leg. Keep the standing leg slightly bent and your stomach in. Neck and shoulders are relaxed. Hips are level. Slide your hands down towards your foot. You should feel the stretch in the muscle between the knee and the hip. Hold for 30 seconds. Repeat four times, alternating legs.

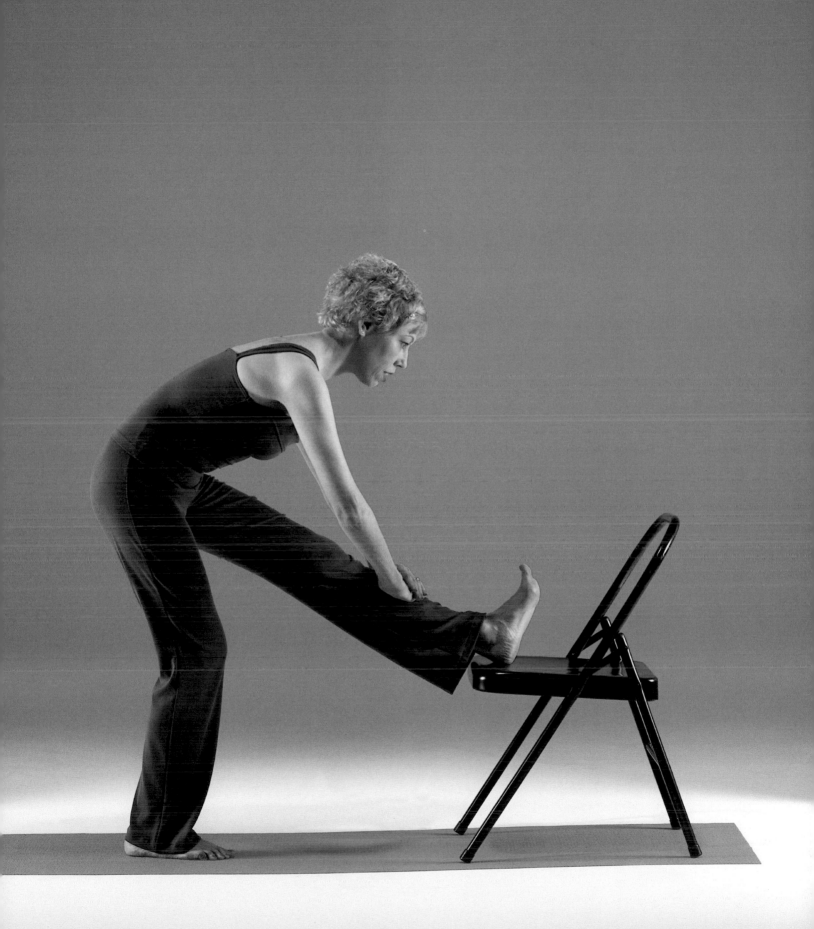

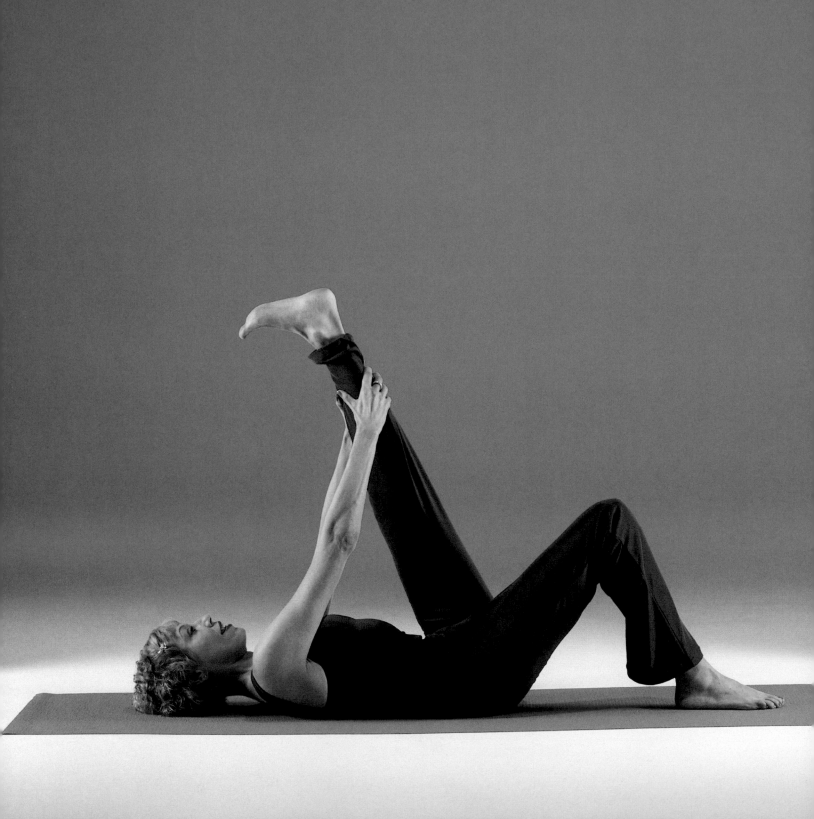

Lying Hamstring Stretch

For this exercise, most people need to place a towel beneath the head. Lie on your mat or towel.

Start with both feet on the floor, making sure you have equal weight down through both feet. The arms are beside you and the pelvis is in the neutral position. Very gently bend your right knee into the chest. Grasp the back of your thigh with your left hand. Grasp the back of your calf with your right hand and gently unfold, straightening that leg with a flexed foot, and ease the leg towards you, moving your left hand up to your calf.

You'll know if you are doing it wrong if your bottom lifts. If this is impossible, instead of using your hands take a towel, place it around your calf and ease the leg towards you, keeping your neck and shoulders relaxed.

Do the right, then the left leg, and repeat, a minimum of twice on each side, holding for 30 seconds.

WATCHPOINT

▷ Don't pull on your leg so that your bottom leaves the floor, as your pelvis will twist. You want to flex the foot without overly tensing the feet, and gently straighten that knee. It is more important to get the knee straighter than to bring the leg closer to you.

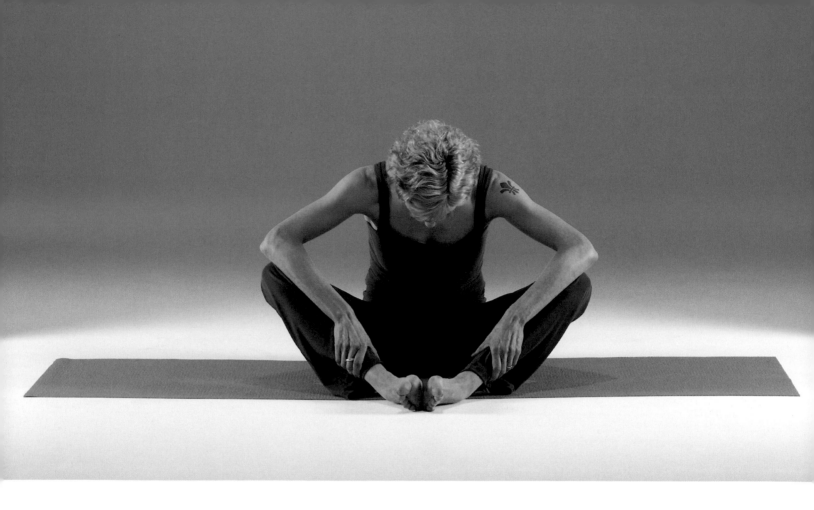

Inner Thigh Stretch

Sit on the floor with the soles of your feet together,
stomach in. Hold onto both ankles. Gently drop your chin
to your chest, relax your shoulders and let your knees
drop to the sides. Hold for 30 seconds. Repeat four
times. If this is difficult, sit on a cushion to begin with.

Advanced Inner Thigh Stretch

Lie on your back, with your legs up a wall. Let your legs
fan out to the sides as far as is comfortable. Make sure
your stomach is in, and your tailbone dropped. If you feel
any pain in your knees, stop. Hold for 30 seconds. Bring
your legs back together. Repeat four times.

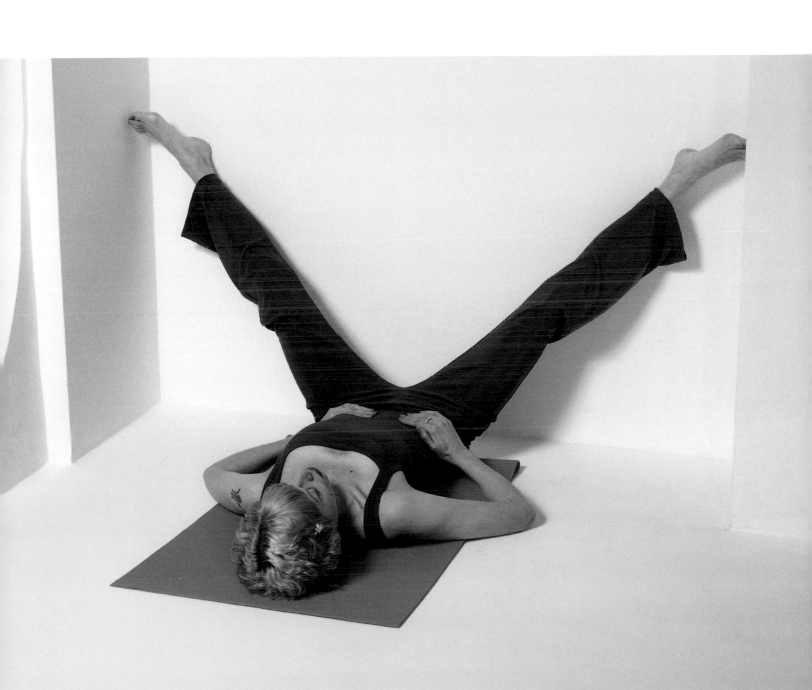

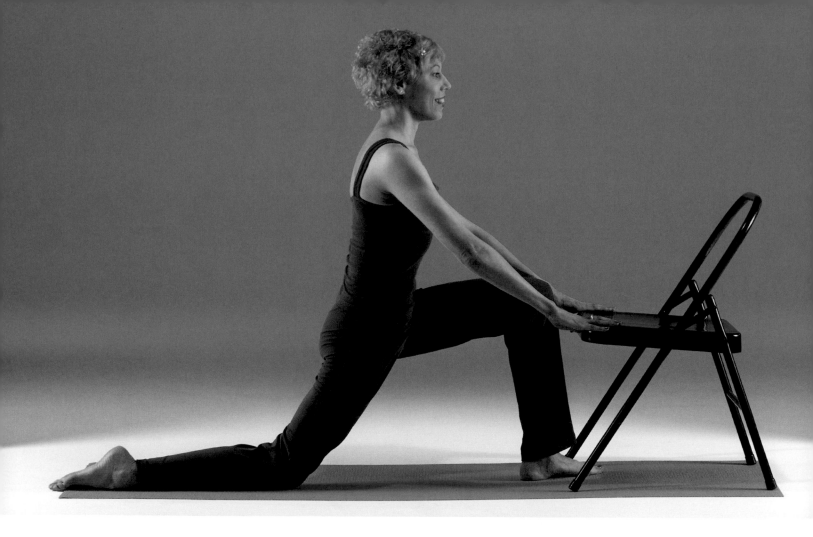

Hip Flexor and Front of the Thigh Exercise

This stretches the front of your thigh, the quadriceps muscle.

Kneeling in a lunge position, holding on to a chair to stabilize your weight, have one foot in front of you with the knee bent. The knee should be directly above the ankle. If the foot is behind the knee, you may strain your knee. You can either have the toes pointing directly forward or at '10 to 2' (think of your foot as a clock hand.) Do whatever feels more comfortable for you. Due to the way in which your lower leg is aligned, the position of comfort may vary. Kneeling on the other leg, the foot behind you, very gently pull your stomach in. Press your hips forward and feel a stretch down the front of the

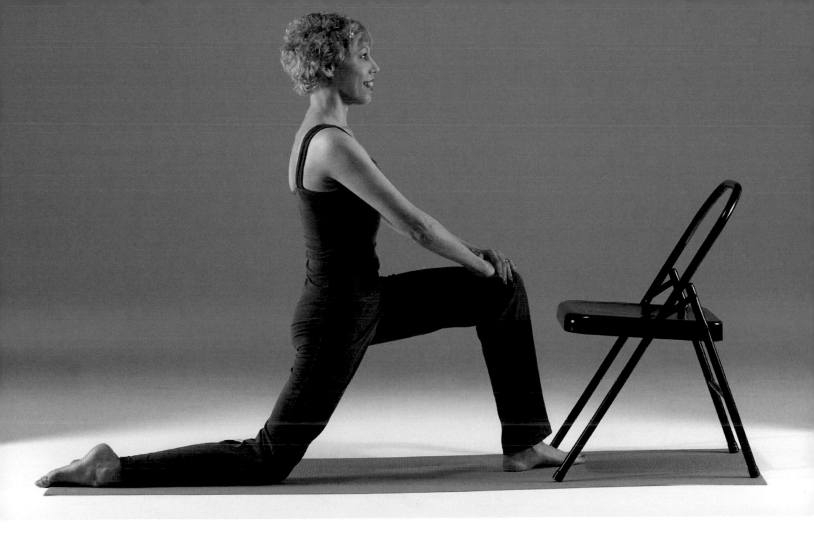

thigh. At no point arch your back. Your stomach is pulled in, your shoulders are relaxed – imagine that someone has one hand on your stomach gently pushing your stomach in and the other hand on your bottom, which is being gently pushed forward to stabilize your spine.

The harder version of this exercise is simply to take your hands away from the chair, put them on your knee and take slightly more of a lean back to get a stronger stretch, but not at the expense of arching your back, straining your knee or letting your stomach protrude.

Repeat the exercise twice on each side, alternating legs.

WATCHPOINT

▷ Don't kneel on a hard floor as you may hurt your knee. With any exercises involving the knees, if you have any knee pain at any time, stop. Pain in the knee is contraindicated in any exercise.

Upper Body

In my experience as a Pilates® teacher, all women want a beautiful upper back, gorgeous shoulders, lovely arms and triceps. The following exercises will tone your back, arms, shoulders and chest. The spine is the central structure of the body. Tight or weak back muscles will eventually lead to problems. Taking steps to strengthen one's back is insurance for the future. A strong back and centre go hand in hand to present an upright and confident person.

You can do second sets when your body builds up to it and follow them with the stretches, which are absolutely essential after performing upper body work. Proper stretching will prevent you from having rounded shoulders and tight muscles.

One combination is press ups, dips and then repeat. An alternative would be a tricep press, bicep curl and then repeat.

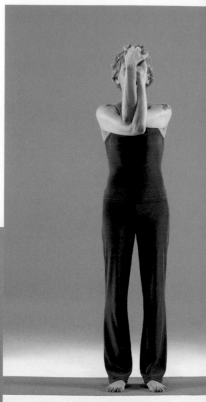

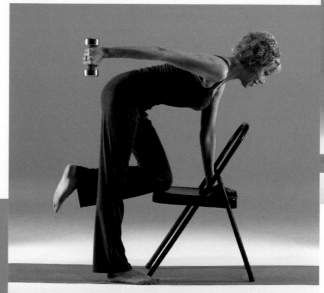

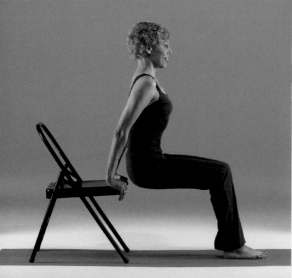

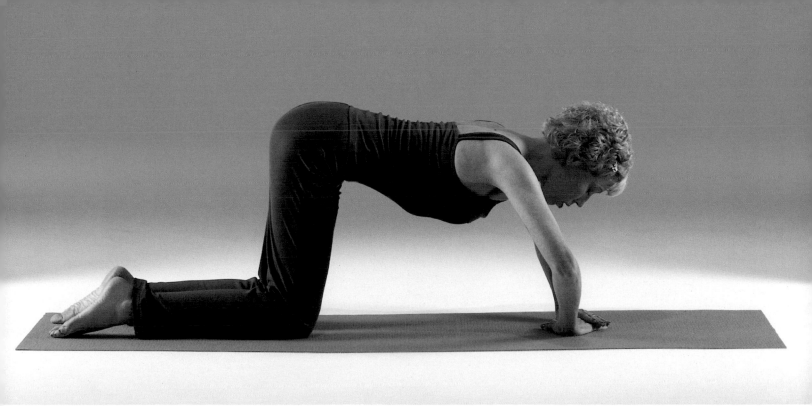

Press-Ups

This exercise is a slight variation of a press-up, which I use a great deal in my studio.

On your hands and knees make a square with the body. Again, it is better not to kneel on a hard surface – use a towel or an exercise mat. To begin, knees are under the hips; the hands are under the shoulders. Cross one hand over the other. The neck is in line. There is no arching the back, the stomach is pulled in. Do not lock the elbows.

In this position, very gently, working with your entire body, tip yourself slightly forward over the arms. This does not mean you should arch your back. It is very natural, when assuming the press-up position, to allow your head to drop. However, try to keep the head in a neutral position, neither forward nor backward.

Begin by doing six repetitions with the right hand on top, then the left. Work up to a set of 10 or 12 with each hand on top. Very gently breathe in as you bend the arms, bringing the chest down. Breathe out as you push away.

If it is possible, do the press-ups in front of a mirror. When you press down, your head should not lower and your chin should not stick out. When you start this exercise you will feel your weight rocking slightly forwards and backwards. Try to stabilize the weight over the arms so that you get the most strengthening through the upper back, the shoulders, the triceps and biceps muscles in the arms. You will be both strengthening and toning. This will not only result in a great-looking upper body, but you will be generating some upper-body strength as well. If you can't easily open your own bottle of champagne, then you have a problem.

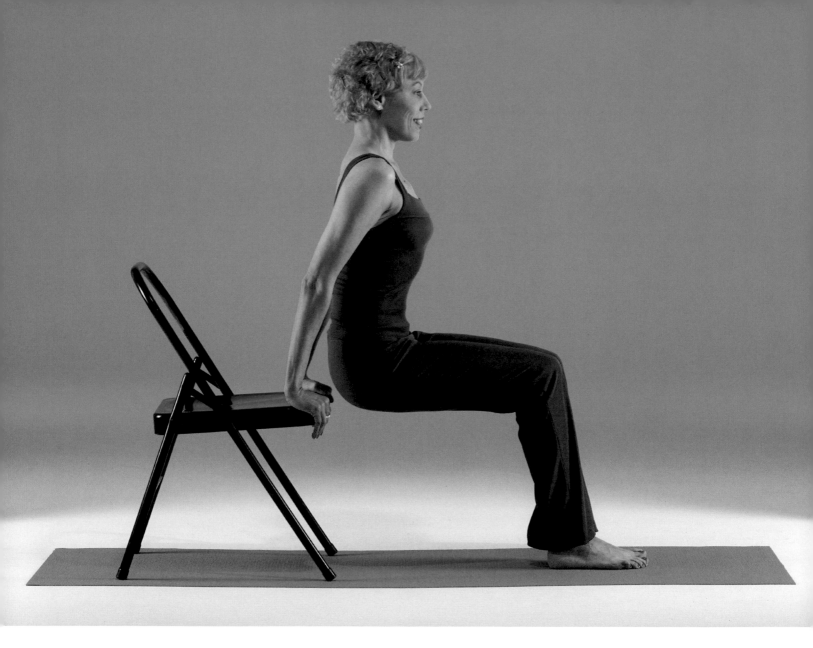

Dips

Most women find dips difficult to start with because of the lack of strength in the backs of their arms.

Using a chair placed against a wall for support, have your hands wide enough so that your shoulders don't feel pinched together. Fingers are facing forward. Make sure in this position that your knees are over your ankles. If they're not you'll be using your thighs as opposed to the backs of your arms. As you breathe in, you bend; as you breathe out, you straighten.

Make sure as you do the dips that you're sliding your

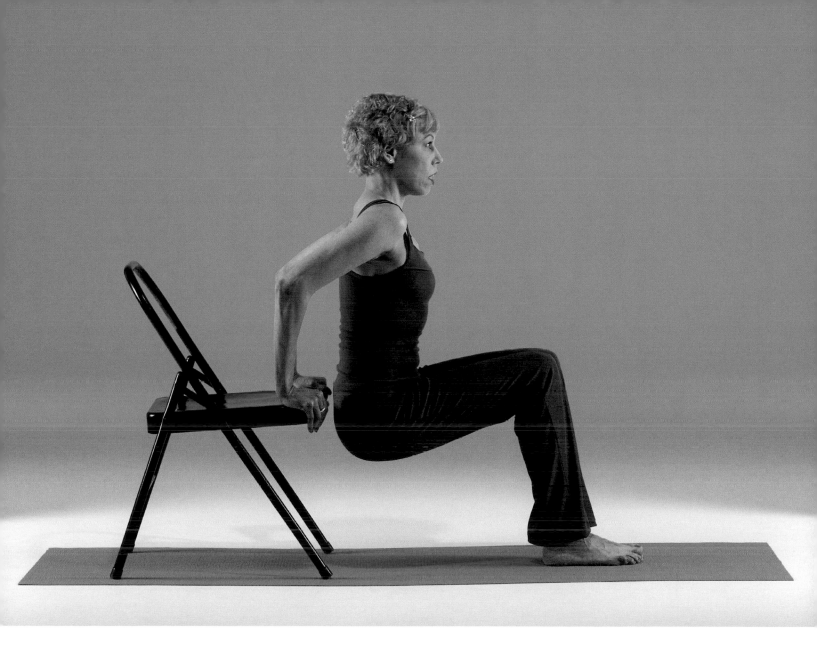

bottom down the edge of the chair and that you're not sliding forward, as the body will automatically prefer to do, and taking the strain in the front of the thighs.

You might only be able to start with eight repetitions; gently build up to 25.

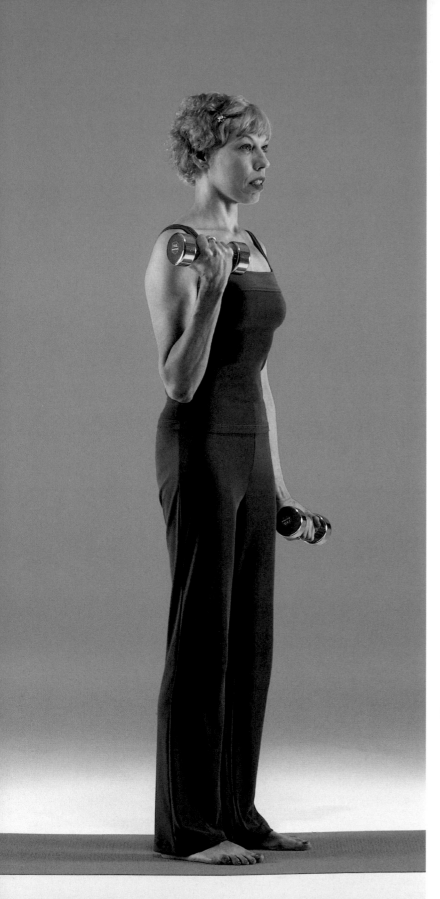

Biceps Curl

Holding a two-kilo weight in each hand, breathe in and bend your arm up to shoulder level. Breathe out and straighten to waist level. Try not to rock as you do this. Repeat 10 to 15 times with alternate arms.

Triceps Press

Using a firm chair, make a square with your body. Place your left hand and knee on the chair, keeping your right leg straight on the ground. Keep your neck in line with the rest of your body. Holding the hand weight, lift your right arm up as high as you can, keeping the elbow bent at a right angle, without twisting the body. Exhale as you straighten the arm behind you. Pause. Bend your arm back again. Repeat 10–15 times on each arm. You may do a second set.

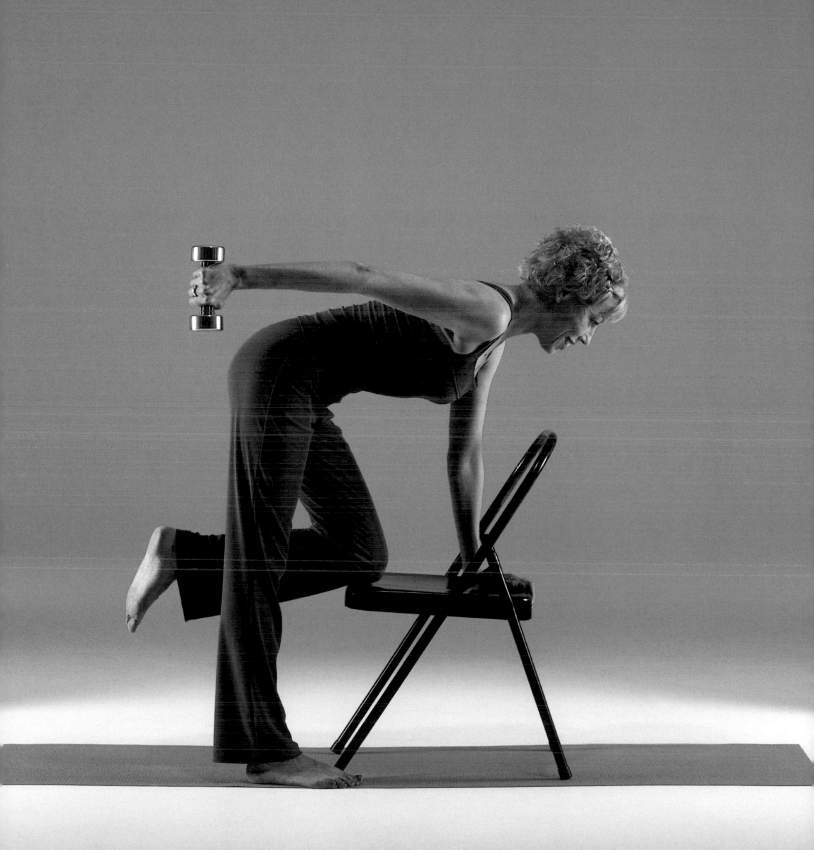

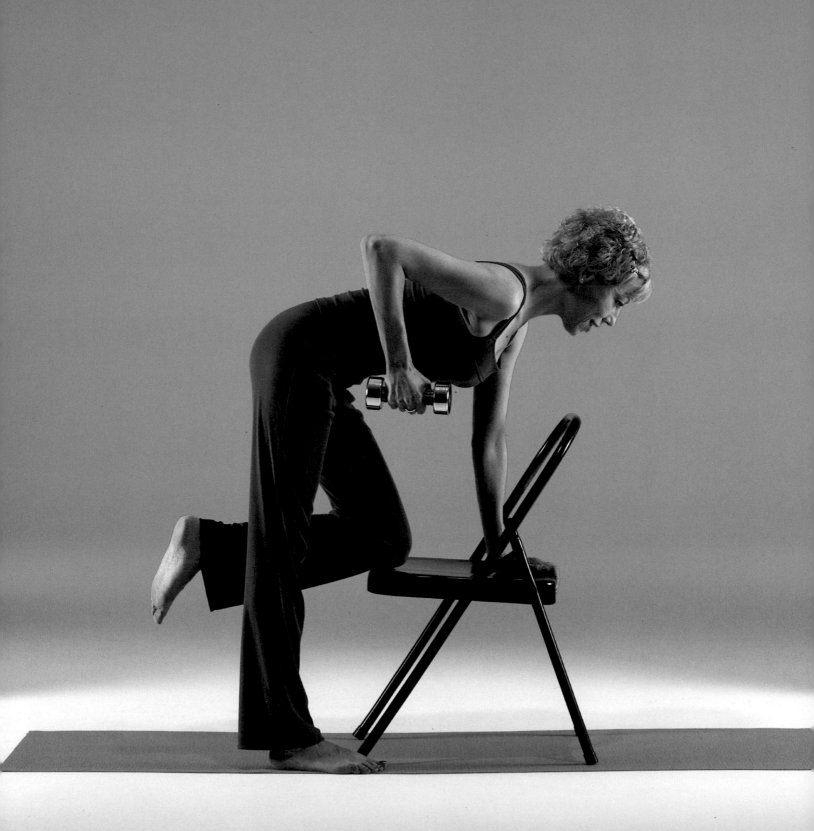

Lat Exercise

Assume the same position as above. (All the same rules apply.) This time you're using your arm to pull up and down. As you 'pull' – feel your lats doing all the work – imagine you're pulling up weeds. Repeat as above.

▷ Do not use your shoulders to do the work in this exercise.

Shoulder Stretch

This stretch can be done seated or standing. Cross one arm over the other and clasp your hands together. Gently push your elbows to the ceiling and feel your shoulders stretching. As you press your arms up, try to keep your shoulders down. Keep your elbows in line with your shoulders. Hold for 10 seconds and then relax. Repeat four times, alternating arms.

▷ If you feel any cramp or discomfort in your shoulders or arms, you are not yet flexible enough to do this.

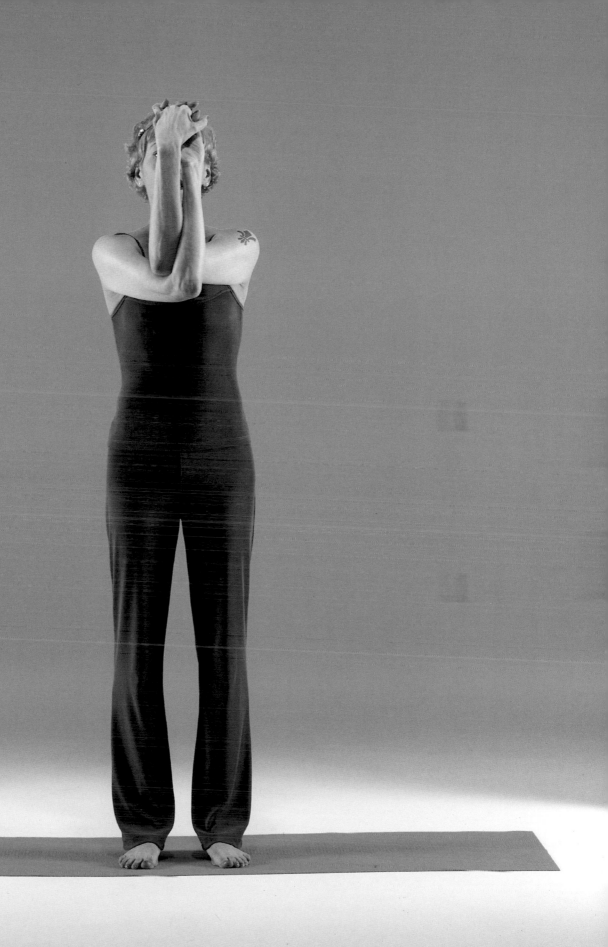

Arms

The following arm exercises are done lying on your back. You should do them after your upper body work. They will help you to keep your shoulders flexible. Place a towel under your head if it feels more comfortable.

In all of these exercises remember to keep your back in a neutral position: don't let your ribs lift. Keep your feet hip-width apart, knees bent, with no tension in the lower back.

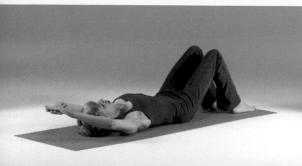

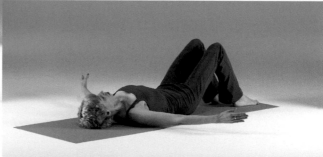

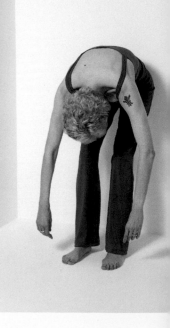

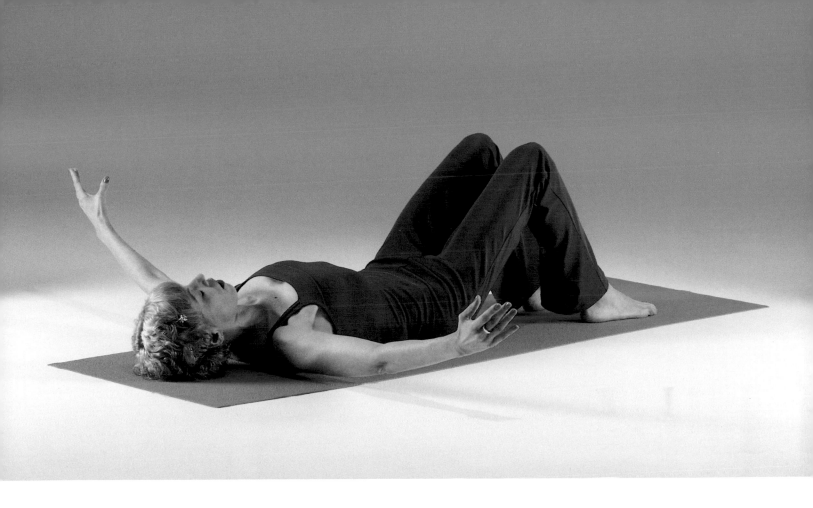

Arms Opening

Lying on your back, raise your arms above your chest
Imagine you're a tulip, and as you breathe out, your arms
gently open. As you breathe in, bring your arms back
together. Keep the curve in the elbows. Repeat 10 times,
opening and closing.

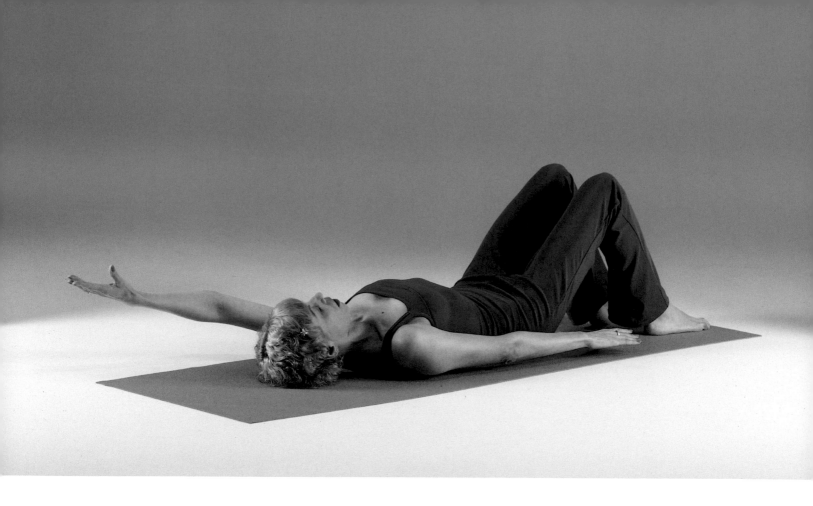

Backstroke

Start in the same position as above. Hold your arms over your chest. The palms face the wall in front of you. Keep your shoulders relaxed. As you breathe out, simultaneously one arm goes down in front of you and one behind you. Breathe in as you reverse the arms. Imagine you're doing the backstroke. Repeat 20 times, 10 on each side.

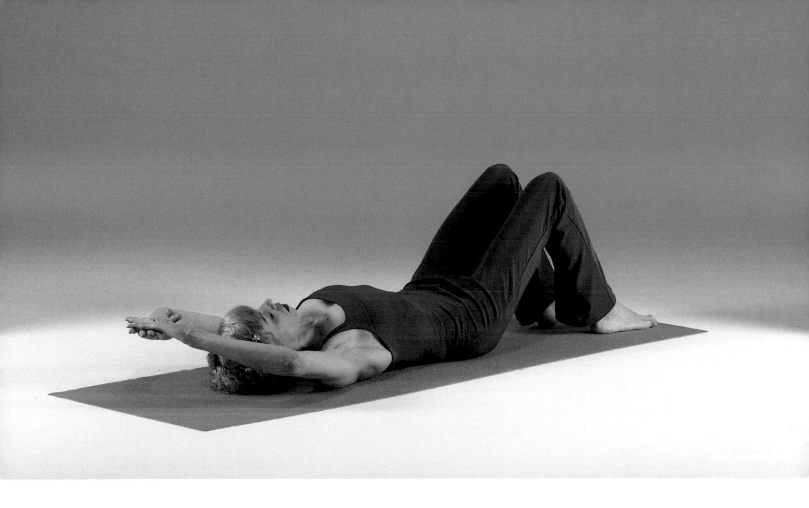

Shoulder Stretch

Assume the same position as in the previous exercise.
Place one hand gently over the other, so that you're
making a diamond shape with your elbows. As you
breathe out, take your arms as far back to the floor, past
your ears, as you can without your back lifting. Repeat
10 times, alternating the hand on top.

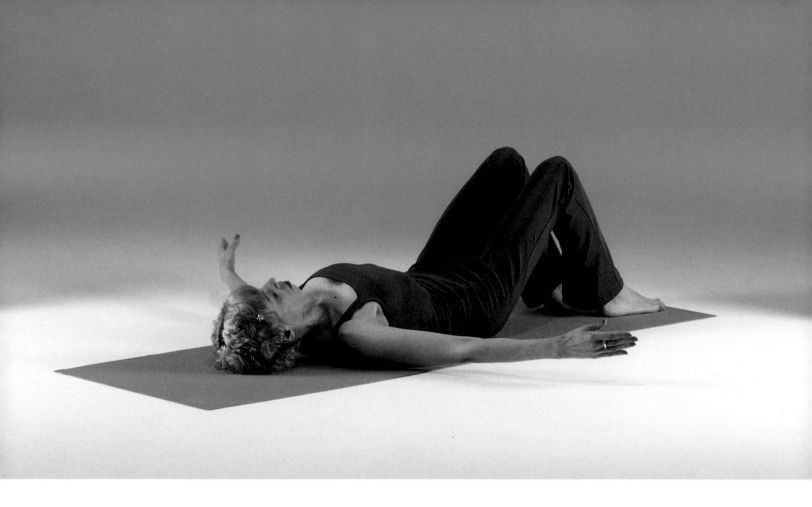

Arm Circles

Assume the same position as in arms opening. With your arms stretched up above you, breathe out and make a circle, so that your hands touch the floor all the way behind you. Bring your arms back and stretch towards your hips. Repeat 10 circles one way and 10 going the other.

To finish

Rolling Up and Down the Wall

This is a great way to relax at the end of any programme, but if you have any back pain don't do this.

Lean your back against a wall. Remember to always keep the knees bent, otherwise you risk straining your back.

Breathe out, and very slowly drop your chin to your chest. It helps if you count as you do this. Start to roll your back down, as gently as you can. By the time you get to a count of eight, your shoulders should roll off the wall. If your legs start to shake, bend your knees a bit more. Roll down as far as you feel comfortable and count for 10–20 seconds. Your arms should now be hanging loosely by your side like a puppet's. Gently move your head from side to side. Pause, and try to roll up, very slowly. Repeat four times (twice down, twice up).

WATCHPOINT

▷ If you've got low blood pressure don't do this, or you might feel faint.

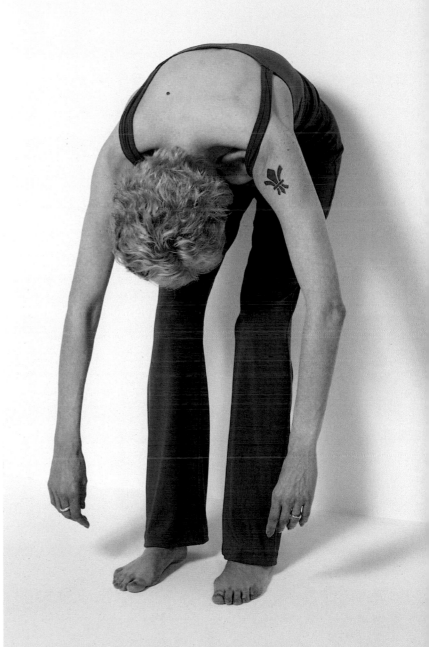

Specific programmes

Lifestyles can create polarization. In other words, we may go from 'living' at the gym to a total abstinence from any form of exercise, the most common reason being lack of time. I have tried to address this problem by weaving these exercises throughout a busy day, making it easier to implement movement during your free time.

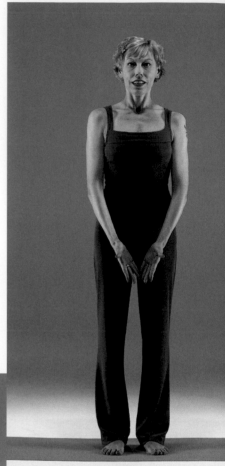

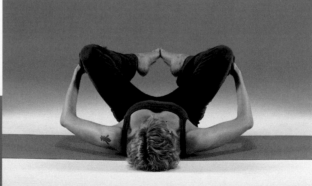

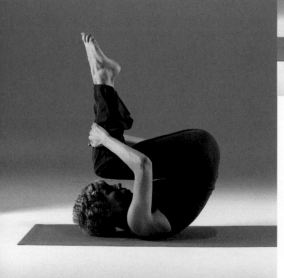

MORNING ENERGIZER

Sleep is supposed to restore us; it is the time when the body regenerates itself. Despite its obviously therapeutic uses, some people don't sleep terribly well. They may have disturbed slumber or they lie in uncomfortable positions.

Often people wake up feeling lethargic, tight and tense. These exercises focus on limbering and release, and will enable you to start your day in a positive frame of mind. Doing these gentle mobilizing exercises early in the day will reconstruct some of the body's internal alignment. This group of six exercises will wake you up, stimulate you and get your joints moving. They will also initiate the feeling of alignment – of standing up straight, feeling balanced and positive.

Exercise Mat or Towel

In all the exercises that involve lying on the floor, it is recommended that you use an exercise mat, but a large bath towel will do. Don't do these exercises on a wooden floor with only a towel. A bath towel placed on a carpet should give enough support to your spine.

Concentrating on limbering and release, this 10-minute programme of morning stretches focuses on releasing the lower spine and hips and gently loosening the upper body. The spine, the upper and lower back and the muscles in the backs of your legs, the hamstrings, will be released. One movement, based on a classic Pilates® exercise, opens up your spine and releases through your discs. Hip rotations will lubricate your hips. The arm exercises will open your shoulder girdle and start getting you to focus on breathing. Finally, there is a side stretch done with a towel to generally stretch and open up. The Morning Energizer should make you feel physical liberation and a spiritual awakening.

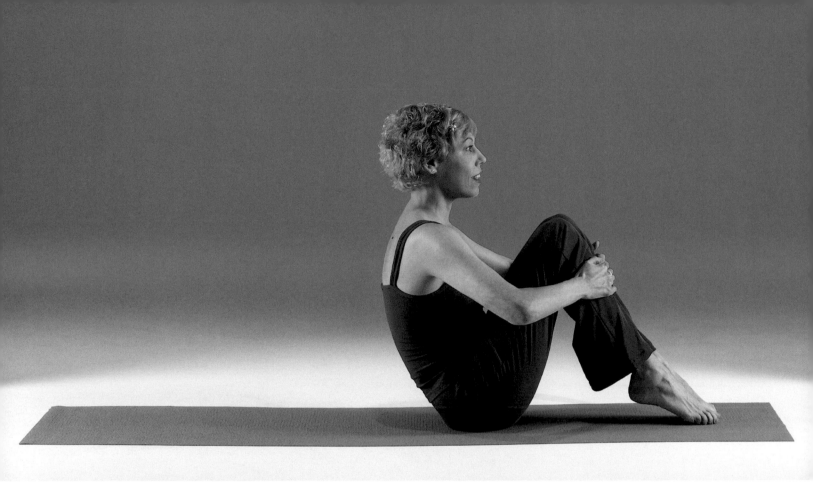

Rolling Up Like a Ball

This exercise can be difficult; work your way into it. Sit holding on to your shins. From the photograph, you can see that I'm curled up like a ball. As you breathe out you roll backwards, and as you breathe in you roll up to a seated position.

Many people don't have a lot of flexibility in the spine, so you might have a problem in getting back up. If this is the case, come back up normally and start the roll again.

Try to keep the heels close to your bottom all the way through, and relax your shoulders. As you breathe out

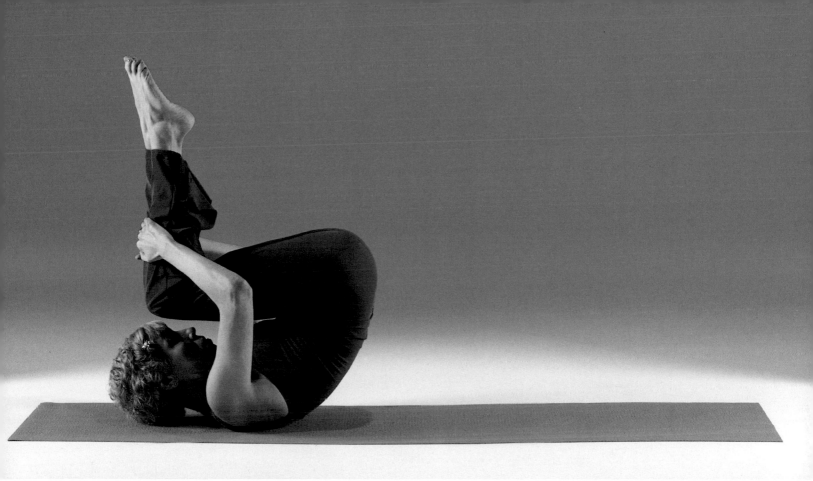

and roll back, the stomach pulls in. Do not roll too high up on the neck. All the exercises are done approximately 10 times. Rolling Up Like a Ball is the exercise I do first when I exercise.

WATCHPOINT

▷ Don't roll too far back onto your neck.

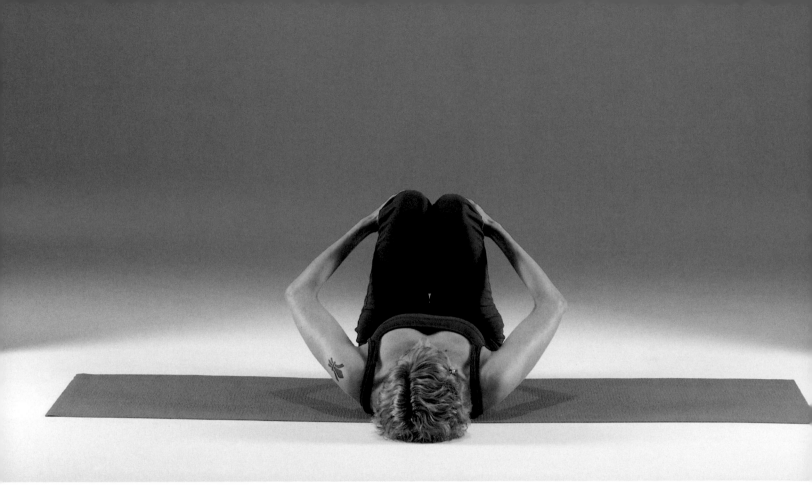

Hip Mobility Exercise

As we get older the hips get tighter, and there is less articulation in the hip socket.

Lie on a large towel or an exercise mat. Keep the feet together and hold on just below the knees. If you feel uncomfortable, put a towel behind your head. The body should not move, the head is resting.

Holding on below the knees, toes together, you rotate your hips 10 times in one direction and 10 times in the other, to lubricate your hips.

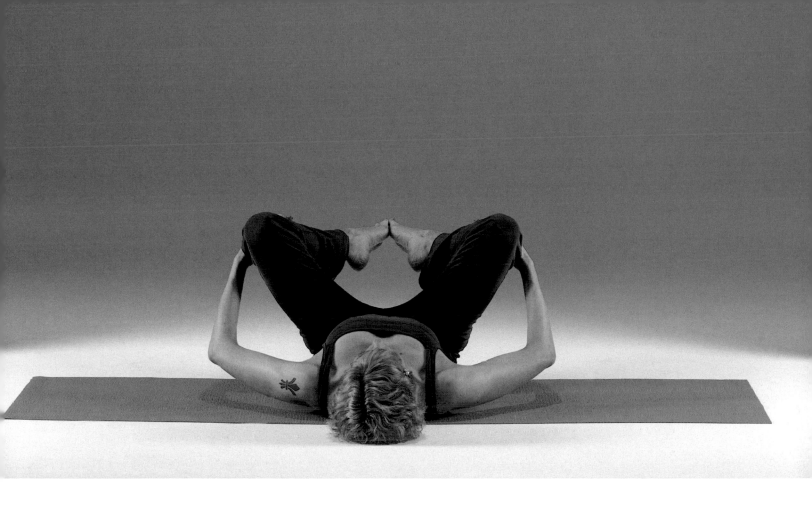

WATCHPOINT

▷ Hold on to your shins and thighs, never the knees.

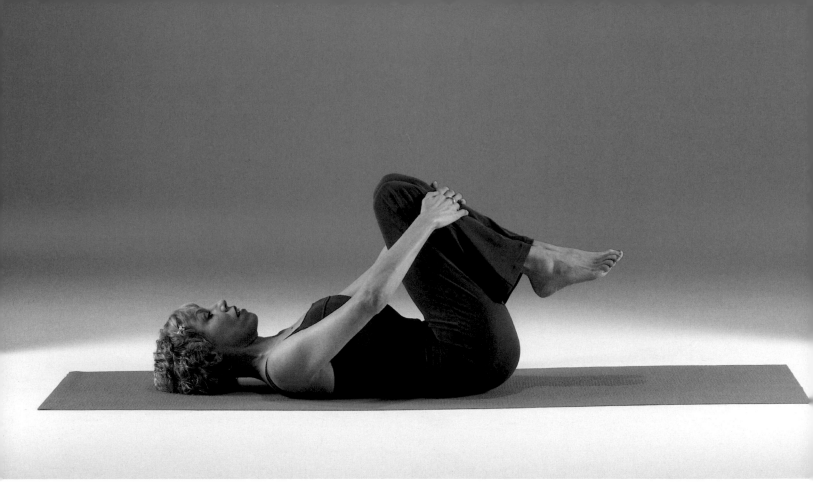

Keeping the toes together, start with the knees apart. As you breathe normally, they come into the chest, then they open and come around. It doesn't matter in which direction you go. This exercise will also help to warm your lumbar spine and the entire pelvis area. You may feel a gentle stretch in your inside thighs if they're tight. Don't force this feeling of stretch. Just feel the mobilization. You're getting blood to flow through your hips and

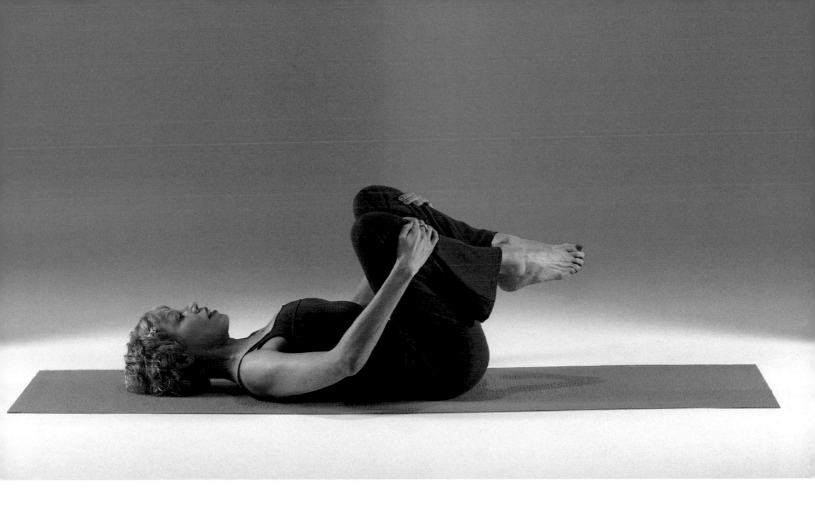

releasing tension through your pelvis. Don't have the legs
too far away from you. Keep the knees over the hips. Your
legs do not hang off your body. Your tailbone is heavy and
supported by the mat or towel at all times.

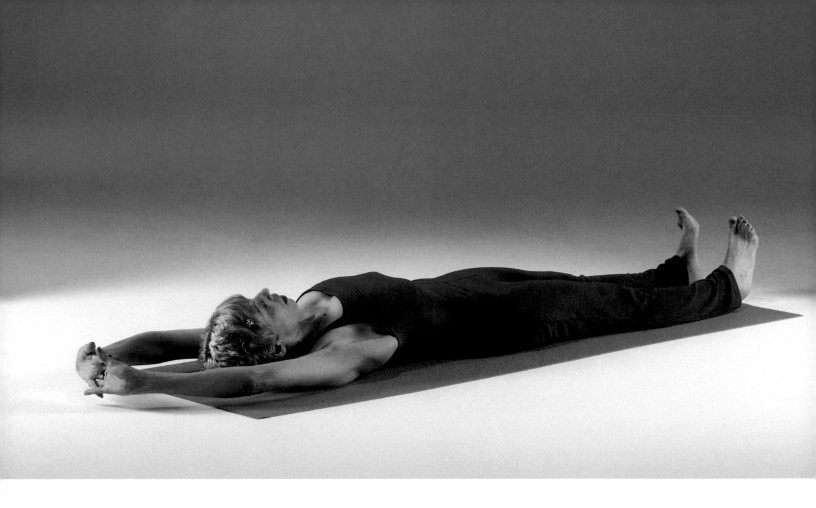

Full-Body Wake-Up Stretch

Lie on your back with a towel behind your head and flex your feet – your toes pointing up towards your knees. Hold your hands, fingers entwined. As you breathe in, the elbows bend so the hands almost touch the crown of the head.

As you breathe out, stretch your arms as far away from you as you can, flex your feet and stretch. Breathe in, bend your elbows, relax, breathe out and stretch. You'll feel this stretch in the back of your legs, your hamstrings, your calf muscles, feet and shoulders. You may feel a stomach stretch as well.

Do approximately 10 repetitions.

You can either do this exercise with the hands crossed or the fingers interlaced. Breathe in, breathe out, and stretch. As you breathe out and stretch, the shoulders shrug up towards the ears. As you breathe in, relax the shoulders, and let them drop. The hands come towards the crown of your head or forehead, the legs relax. As you breathe out, the fingers and hands stretch away, the shoulders lift, the feet stretch towards the other end of the room with flexed feet. The body is stretched and energized.

Warm-Ups for Shoulders and Back

These two exercises are about postural awareness. At this point do not stand on a towel unless you feel very secure. This exercise is better done with bare feet, so you can feel the contact with the floor.

Stand with your feet hip-width apart. Relax your feet. Make sure the weight is evenly placed over your feet, try not to sink either forward or backward. The toes are relaxed and lengthened as if they're softening into sand. When you're standing upright the stomach is gently pulled in, the tailbone drops, the pelvis is in neutral. You're not gripping your hamstrings or the back or front of your legs.

Start with the arms naturally relaxed at your side. They don't hang behind you, they gently soften, as if your middle finger is stretching down the outside of your thigh, lengthening away. In this position the hands are just in front of you. The shoulders are relaxed and the head is in a neutral position. Don't let your head drop forward or back. Let it sit on top of your shoulders. Use visualization techniques and think of your head as a blossom sitting on the stem of a plant. The head is just softly there. The knees are released.

The first exercise is very simple. Begin with the arms beside you. As you breathe out, one arm reaches to the ceiling, and the other arm gently reaches to the wall behind you without any shift in the feet, the pelvis, the upper back or the neck. If you're feeling that shift you are taking the movement too far for your initial flexibility. This exercise can be done either 10 times, 5 on each side, or 20, which is 10 on each side, alternating the arms.

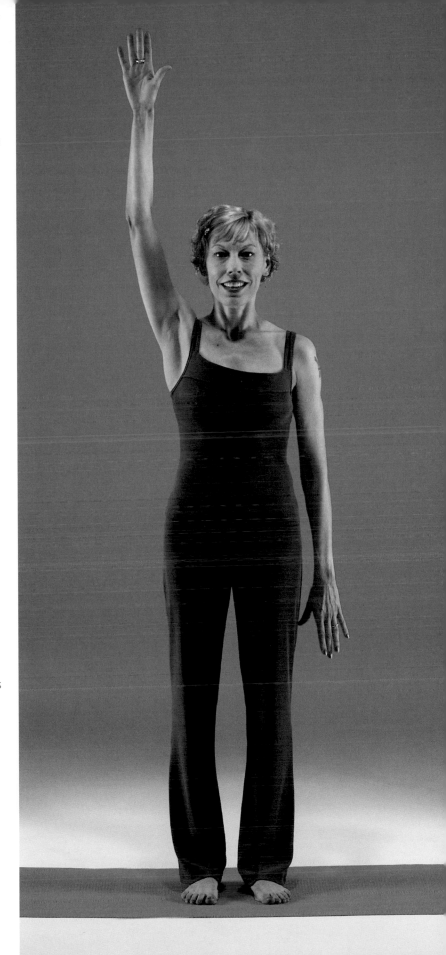

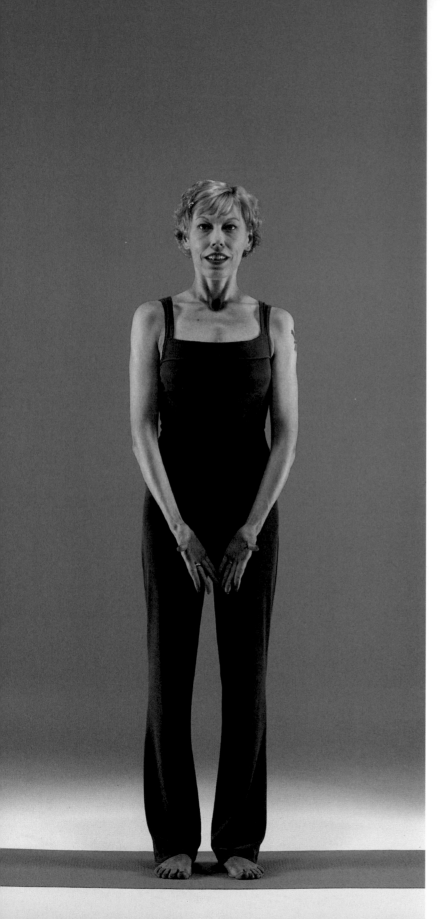

The second exercise targets the same area. Start with the same postural alignment, no gripping of the feet, no tensing of the buttocks – everything is relaxed and calm. Straighten both your arms and bring them in front of you with the tips of the little fingers touching.

As you breathe out, take a slice and reach to the corners of the room. The arms stay straight all the way through. Breathe in, breathe out, then slice, reaching for the corners of the room.

WATCHPOINT

▷ With any of the arm exercises, at no point do you lock your elbows. The joints are in line: the shoulders, the elbows, the wrist, all the fingers – don't break at the wrist.

After you've done this second exercise 10 times you may do a few on the diagonal. You slice, gently twist and the head follows. You will feel a gentle stretch across the chest and some stretching through the shoulders.

These exercises are also about coordination. In the first exercise both arms work rhythmically, alternating. In the second exercise you want both arms to start and end at the same point. You don't want one arm to begin before the other.

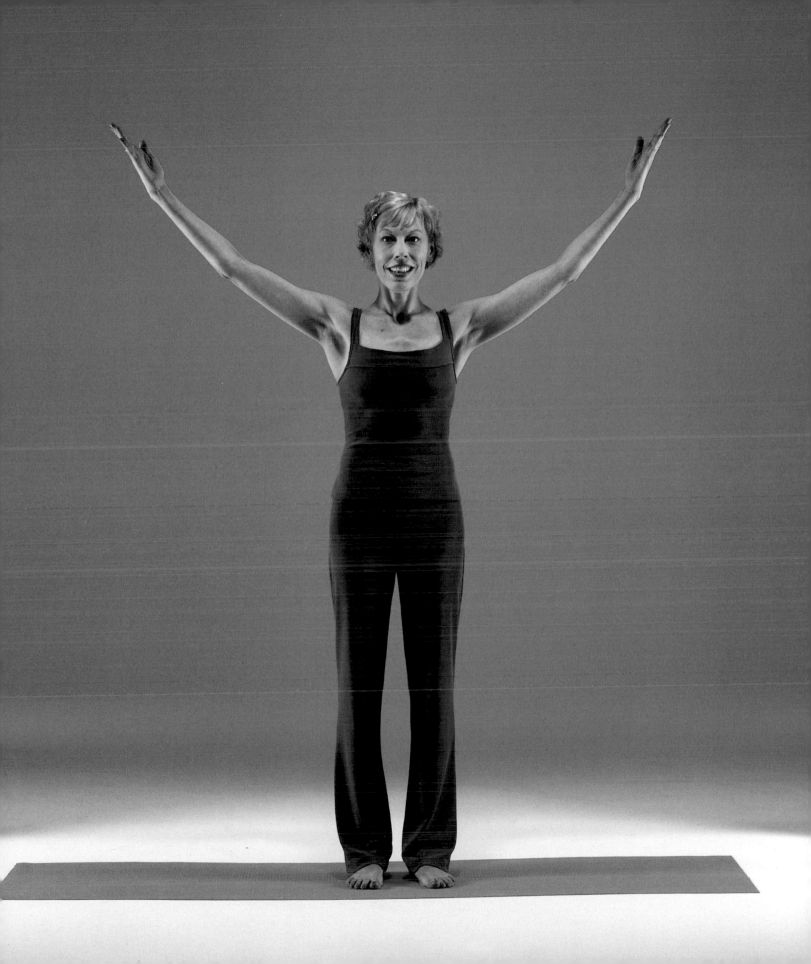

Waist Stretch

Stand in the same position, holding a folded hand towel nice and wide between your arms. Breathe out, stretch to one side. Breathe in, straighten up, and breathe out to stretch to the other side. Don't lift your shoulders up to your ears, and stretch only as far as you don't shorten on the underneath side.

Your weight should be evenly balanced over both feet. You'll know you've gone too far if you feel one foot coming off the floor. The weight is over the second toe, as in all of the standing exercises. Hips don't move very much because it is a waist-energizing stretch. Breathe out as you take the stretch, breathe into the centre and breathe out as you change.

Do approximately 10 repetitions on each side.

The waist stretch is related to core strength. You engage your abdominals to stabilize your pelvis and your spine during a gentle waist stretch; the body does not collapse from side to side.

WATCHPOINT

▷ Keep the weight evenly distributed over both feet for the duration of the exercise and don't allow yourself to tip from one side to the other.

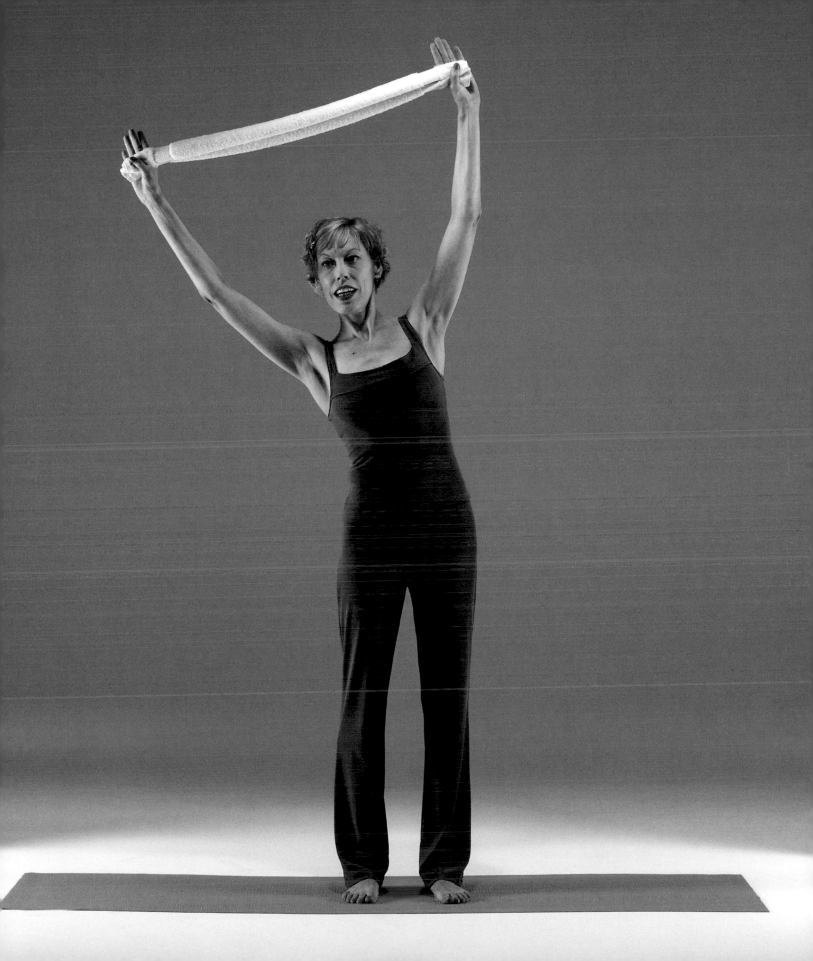

Integrated Postural Awareness at Work

With these exercises you will maximize posture and energy levels in environmentally unfriendly conditions. You will learn to sit and stand correctly throughout the day. New habits will form and, once learned, will be hard to break. Your body will feel comfortable and well-balanced, freeing you to be mentally alert.

Generally people sit badly. They sink into their hips when they sit down. Most people are not as active as they should be because of the restrictions in their daily lives. These exercises will take you back to basics,

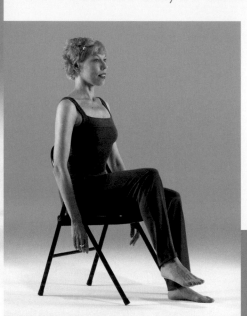

re-creating the way you sit. The emphasis in these exercises is not on complicated movement but on visualization.

You are sitting at your desk, with your chair at the right level, with your feet grounded through the floor, and equal pressure down through both feet. Your lower back is supported in the chair, the upper back floating above with no tension. A shoulder stretch has also been included, which will release tense shoulders. You then breathe into your stomach and, on the exhale, you contract your stomach into the back of the chair, concentrating on feeling that movement of internal support as you grow taller and more confident.

Sitting Properly

Sit with your back supported by a chair. Your tailbone is heavy, both feet are evenly placed on the floor. You are in contact from your centre directly down through your feet into the floor. You're going to channel your energies from your centre out through the crown of your head. Your shoulders are relaxed, your arms are relaxed because your middle back is supported. Your tailbone will drop and your abdominals will naturally pull back towards your spine. Again, try to think of your head sitting naturally on top of your shoulders, not pushing forward and not pushing back.

WATCHPOINT

▷ If you force your shoulders back and your lower back arches away from the chair, you know your shoulders are still too rounded for you to maintain this position and be anatomically correct.

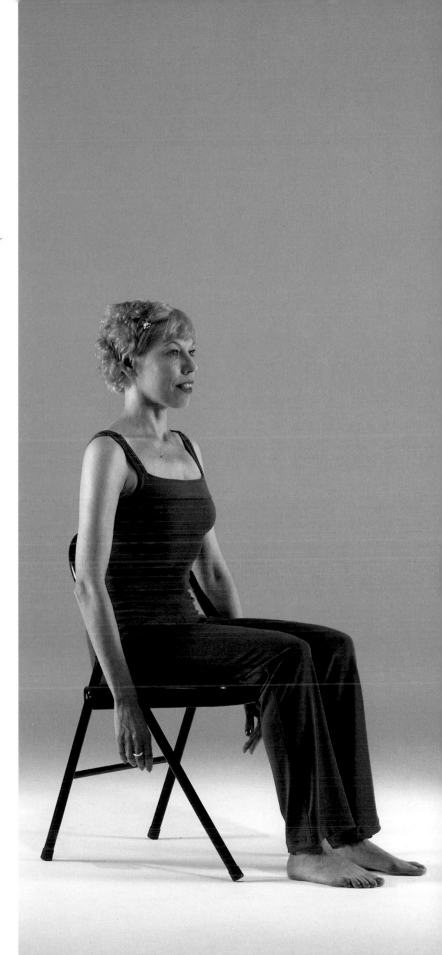

Breathing

Starting with this basic seated position, place your fingers on your lower abdominals, the space between your pubic bone and your navel. As you breathe in the stomach gently expands, filling with oxygen. As you breathe out the stomach pulls away from your fingers and settles back into the chair, your navel pulls away from your fingers and you feel the energy going in to support the lower back. Repeat 10 times.

Foot Lifts

You can either have your fingers on your abdomen in the same place as the previous exercise or allow your arms to hang naturally beside you. As you breathe in your abdomen gently softens or expands into your fingers, as you breathe out you very gently let one foot float off the floor, feeling the connection of the navel to the spine. Place the foot down, make sure you have even pressure through both feet again, and change legs. The coordination is important. Start off foot lifts very slowly; eventually you will be able to do them faster so the interchange emanates from a stable pelvis and a strong abdomen.

Initially the change from one leg to the other might feel unstable as you don't have the core strength to coordinate alternate leg lifts automatically. The feet should float off the floor. Do 10 lifts with each leg, alternating each time.

WATCHPOINT

▷ If you lift your feet too high, you will feel your pelvis sink back into the chair and you'll lose that postural alignment. Your tailbone will tuck underneath and your back will curl.

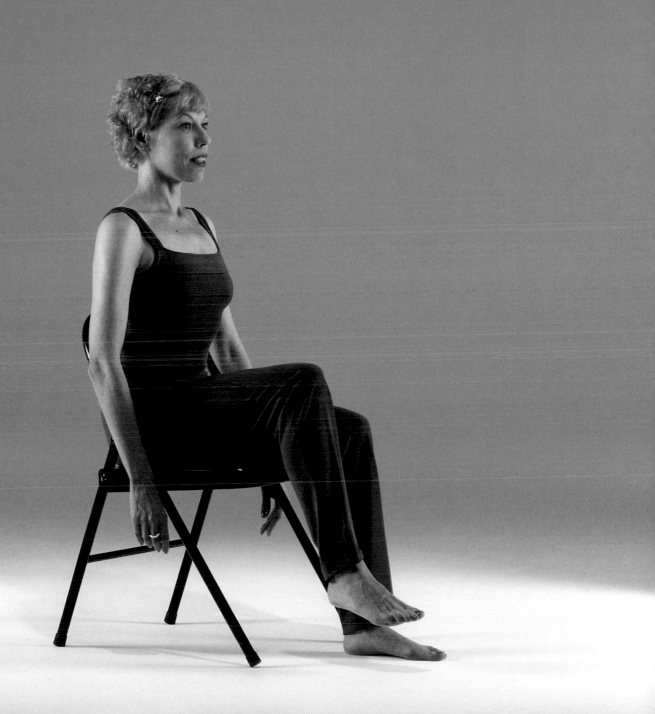

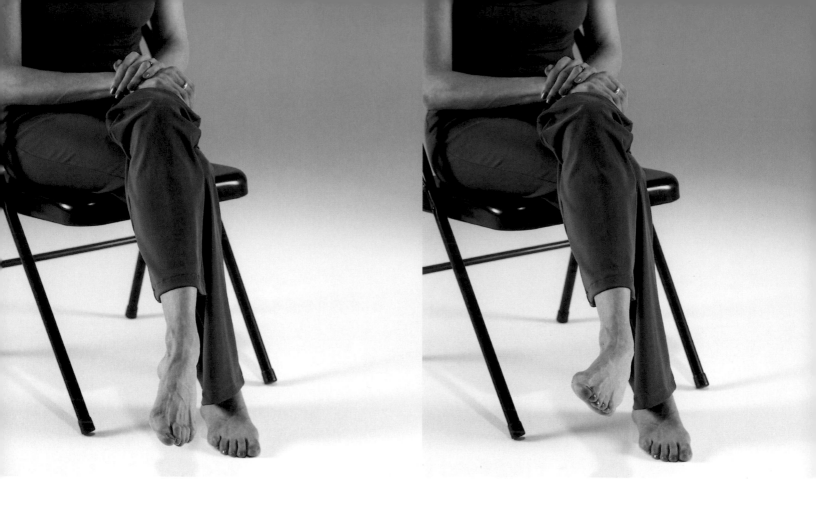

Relax Your Ankles

This exercise will relax your ankle, calf and foot, and it will give you a conscious feeling of the connection between your body and the earth.

Slip your shoes off, cross one knee over the other and gently circle your ankle very slowly, so that you take six seconds to circle the ankle in one direction, approximately six to eight times. Change directions and repeat, then do the same thing with the other ankle.

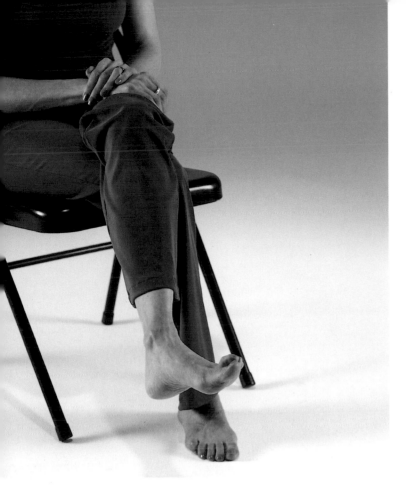

WATCHPOINT

▷ Try to keep your toes relaxed, don't grip with
  your toes. Do not move the bones in your lower leg
  (the tibia and fibula). Think of your ankle bones as
  pebbles that you're gently shaking. As you're
  circling the ankle, the pebbles are lubricating and
  relaxing. If you tense your foot and lower leg, this
  won't happen. Your ankle and calf will feel warmer
  after this exercise, if completed slowly and
  rhythmically.

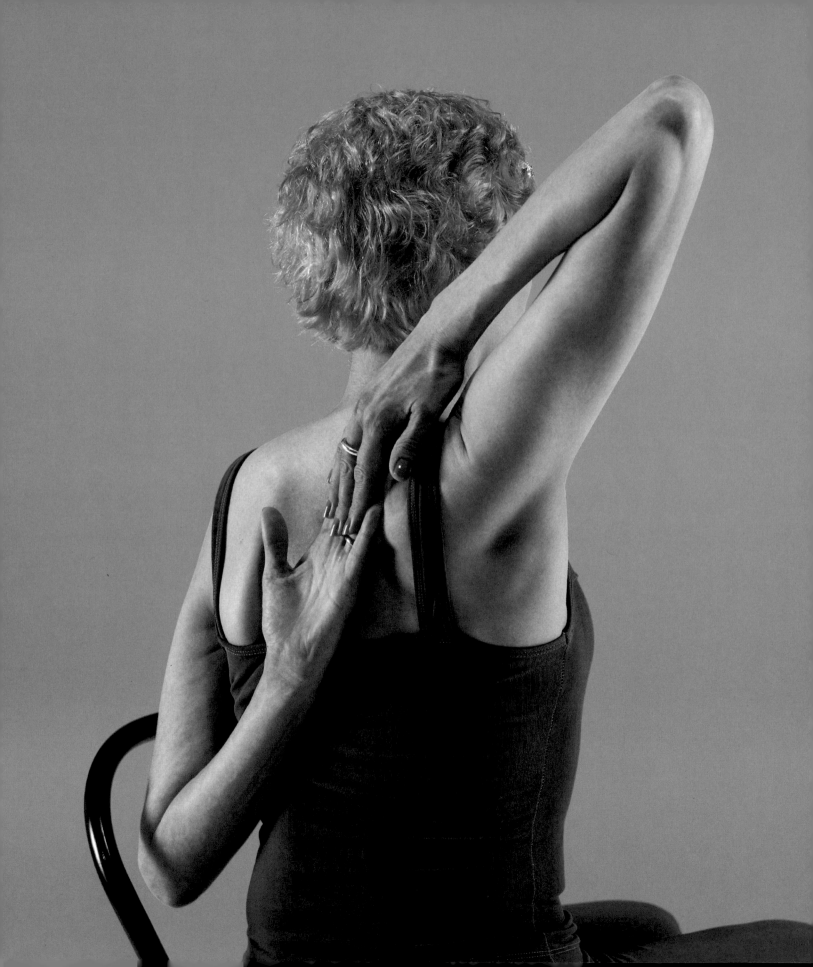

Shoulder Stretch

Seated in your chair, all the above rules apply: stomach pulled in, tailbone dropped, both feet evenly balanced on the floor. Think of your energy evenly placed down through both feet. Very gently, take your right hand and place it on your left shoulder blade, palm facing down. Take your other hand and try to reach and connect your fingers behind you. If you can't do this initially, don't worry, aim to do it eventually. Without arching your back or sticking your chest out, gently open out the right or the left top arm to stretch. Keep the neck long. Do the other side, then approximately five times on each side, alternating sides.

Neck Stretch

This neck stretch should not be done more than four times.

Sitting in your chair, gently place the palm of your hand not on your neck, but behind the crown of your head.

Sit with your feet comfortably apart, drop your chin towards your chest without leaning forward, look at your big toe and gently press your head against your hand; feel the neck stretching. Hold for 20 seconds. Relax, do the stretch on the left and once more on either side.

WATCHPOINT

▷ Middle back should be supported, tailbone dropped; don't let the chin go forward.

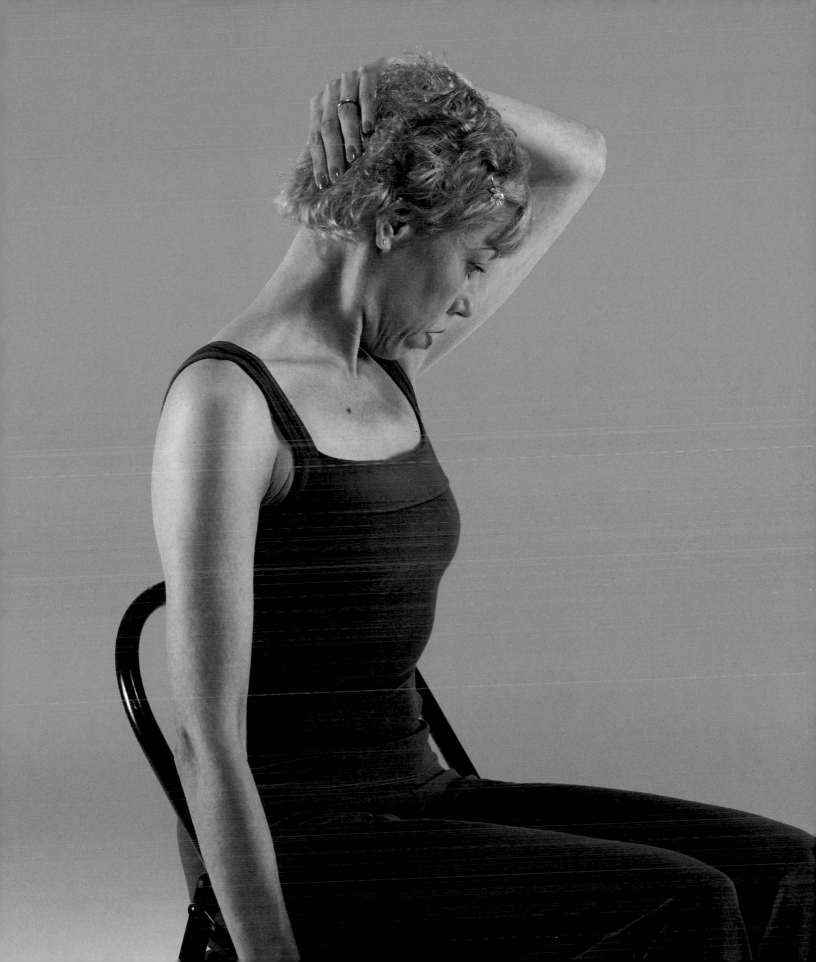

Midday Break

The human mind and body don't function at their best after working for eight consecutive hours. You need to have a space or break in your working day, whether it's a brisk walk or reading a newspaper. A change of environment – physical or mental – will recharge your batteries. Your mind and body will be clearer and you'll feel less sluggish in your working environment.

An active aerobic break combined with stretches and body-releasing exercises makes a lunch break a good time to rejuvenate and recharge. 'Aerobic' is a very general term that can indicate anything from climbing the stairs to taking a short walk.

This programme is a restart and refocus. It involves a lot of stretching. It will address the areas that are tight from sitting and working, and will be especially helpful for those who work in front of a computer screen.

You will stand up and do some very simple foot exercises, such as grasping the floor with your toes and releasing, followed by calf stretches, a shoulder stretch and a cat stretch. There is also a stretch in which you stand in the doorway and release your shoulders. This focuses the energy away from areas of work-induced tightness so you can feel relaxed and liberated when you lunch. You can then enjoy your lunch break, as you will have rid yourself of work-related muscular stress.

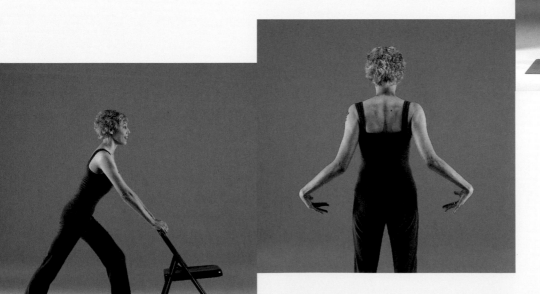

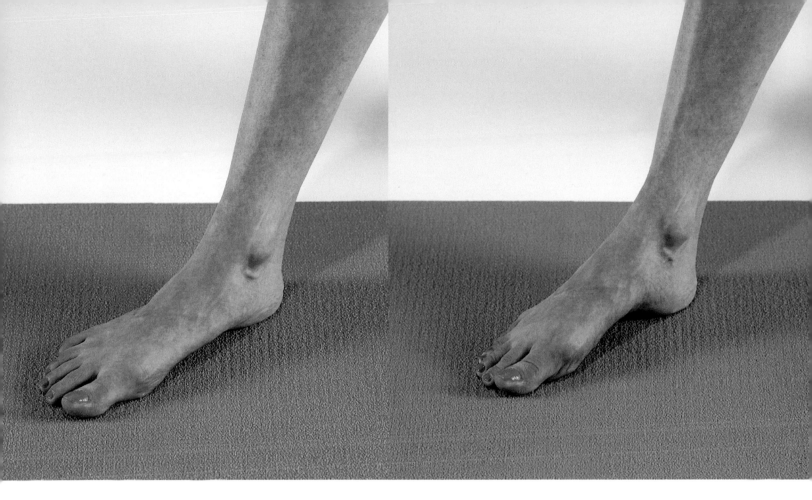

Doming

Doming is better done with bare feet. Very gently lift your foot so that you're just resting on your heel. As you place your foot on the ground, spread your toes and try to separate them. Ideally they will all spread and separate at the same time. (Imagine doing doming with your hand: you lift and separate your fingers as you place them down.)

Holding your toes down, you draw up the arch underneath your foot, without gripping your toes. Relax. As you flex onto the heel and spread the toes, imagine having chewing gum under the ball of your foot. You draw your toes up – without gripping the floor – and relax. In the beginning you might get cramp in your foot. Do 10 repetitions with each foot.

WATCHPOINT

▷ Do not let your toes become 'clawed'.

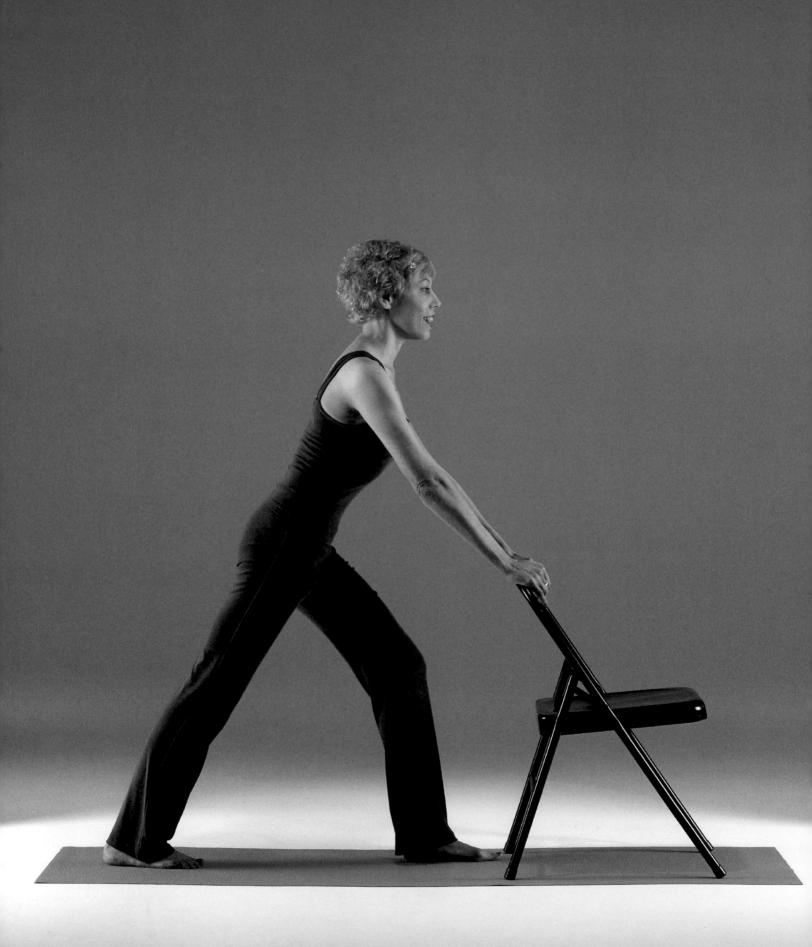

Calf Stretch

Again, this exercise is done without shoes. Using your office desk or chair, take a very simple calf stretch. Shoulders are down, the stomach is in, the tailbone dropped. Don't arch your back or stick out your ribs. Keep your shoulders down and the head floating on top of your body. Have both feet hip-width apart, take a step forward with one leg and feel a stretch down the back of the other, the heel touching the floor. Hold for 30 seconds, then do the other leg. Repeat again.

WATCHPOINT

▷ Stomach in, tailbone dropped.

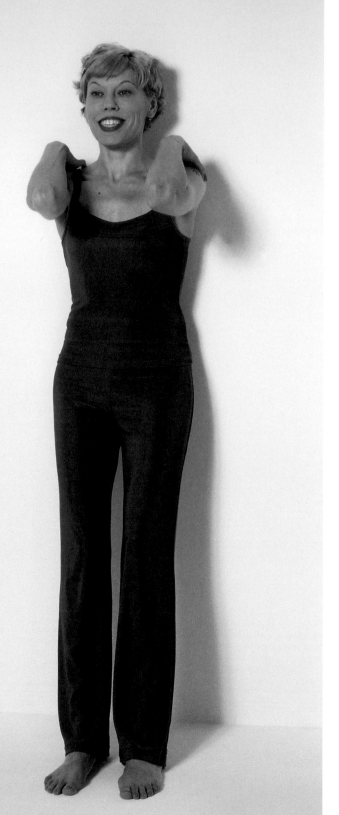

Shoulder Rotation

This exercise will open up your shoulders. It can be done seated in an office chair, but the preferred position is against a door frame or wall.

Lean with your knees bent and middle back against the wall, and slide down, keeping the knees bent. Your weight is placed evenly over the feet, which are not tense. Your middle back and the space between your shoulder blades touch the wall for support. Do not push your head back as you will feel your middle back and shoulder blades come off the wall.

WATCHPOINT

▷ Keep your middle back and the space between the shoulder blades on the wall.

Breathing normally, gently place your hands on your shoulders. This exercise consists of four movements: circle arms forward, trying to get the elbows to touch, lift up towards the ears, circle as far back as you can without any of your middle back coming off the wall. When you have completed the movement, you then circle the other way. Back, up, around and down. Do 10 repetitions in each direction.

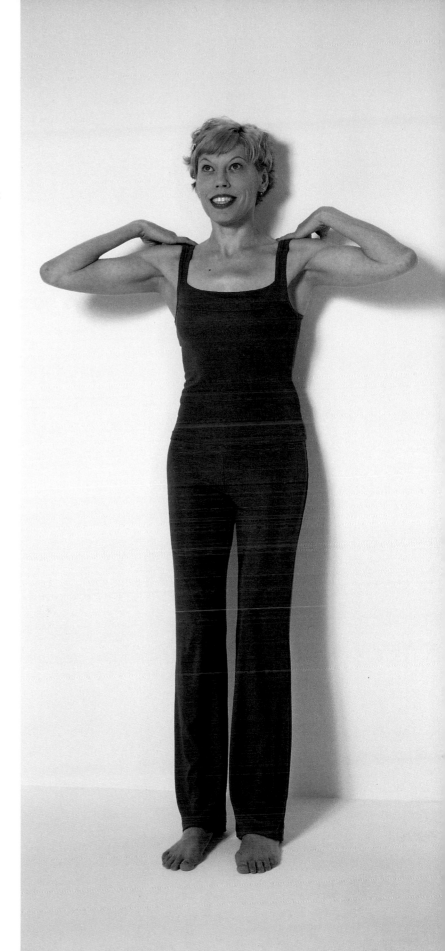

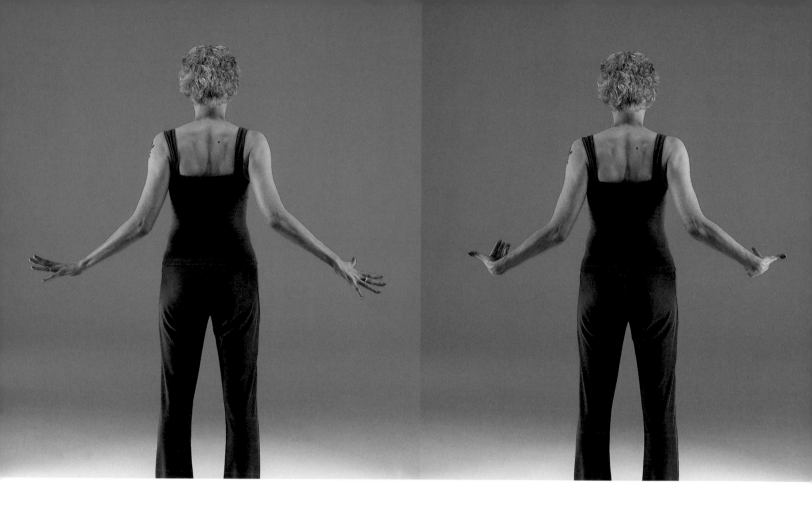

Hand Exercises

The next two exercises will help those with stiff hands or people suffering from Repetitive Strain Injury.

Sit or stand with your shoulders relaxed. Stretch your hands very gently and bring each finger to the thumb, beginning with the little finger. Stretch each of your fingers as much as you can.

You can either do this exercise with your hands in front of you or behind you. The movement is exactly the same, but in this instance you circle the wrist. Think of Balinese dancers. This exercise also works on coordination.

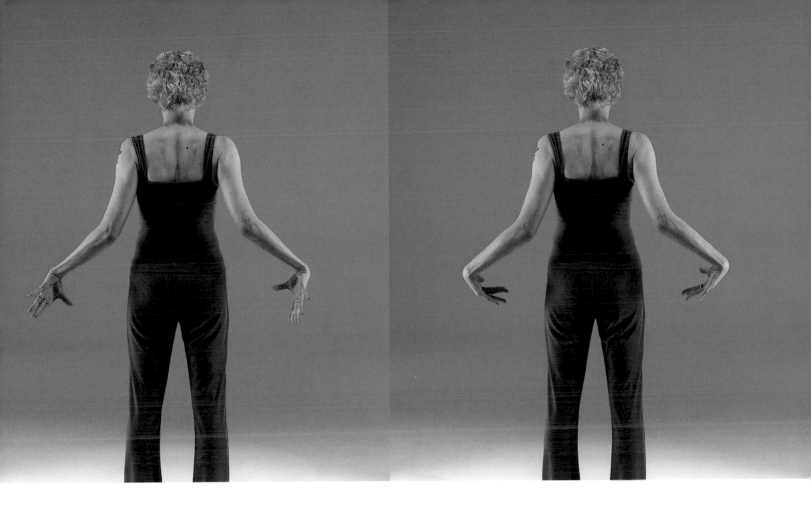

▷ Keep the shoulders and elbows relaxed.

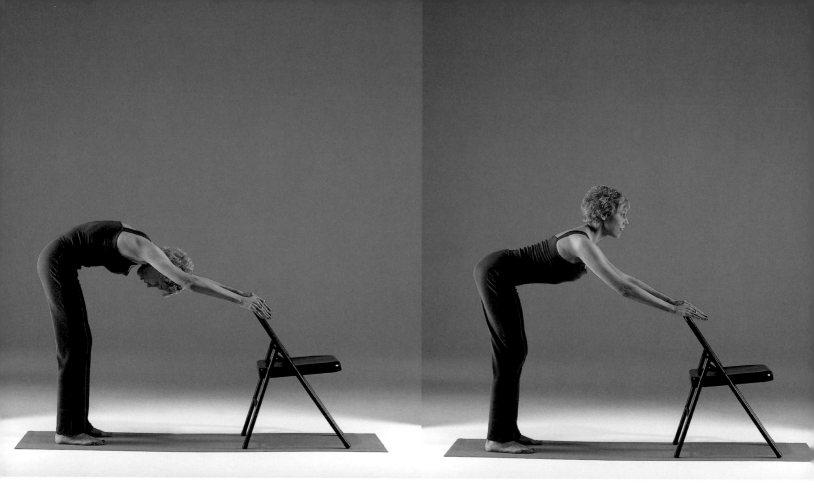

Cat Stretch at the Desk

Using an office desk or chair, this exercise will release
your lower back and stretch out your shoulders. Shoes
are off unless you're in flat shoes. Do not do this exercise
in heels.

Stand as far away from your desk as you can while still
resting your palms on the desk. Bend your knees slightly
and keep them bent. Weight goes down evenly through
both feet.

Breathe out, curl your chin into your chest, your
stomach into your spine. Stretch out your lower back.
This will counteract the effects of being seated for long
periods of time, and get the blood flowing as you open
your spine.

As you breathe in, press your chest down; your bottom
goes up and the head gently lengthens back.

WATCHPOINT

▷ If you feel the neck crunching or your vocal cords
contracting you've taken your head too far back.
There should be no discomfort in your neck.

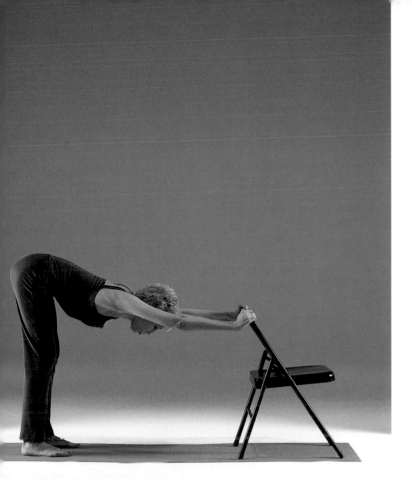

Shoulder Stretch

Again, stand as far away from your desk as you can
with your palms resting on it. Bend your knees slightly
and keep them bent. Weight goes down evenly through
both feet.

For this shoulder stretch keep the ears between the
arms. Holding on to the desk, press your chest down and
stretch your arms to give your shoulders, neck and upper
arms a good stretch. Don't worry if you feel a little ache in
your upper arms, because it is 'referred pain' from
stretching out your upper back.

WATCHPOINT

▷ Keep knees bent and head between the arms.

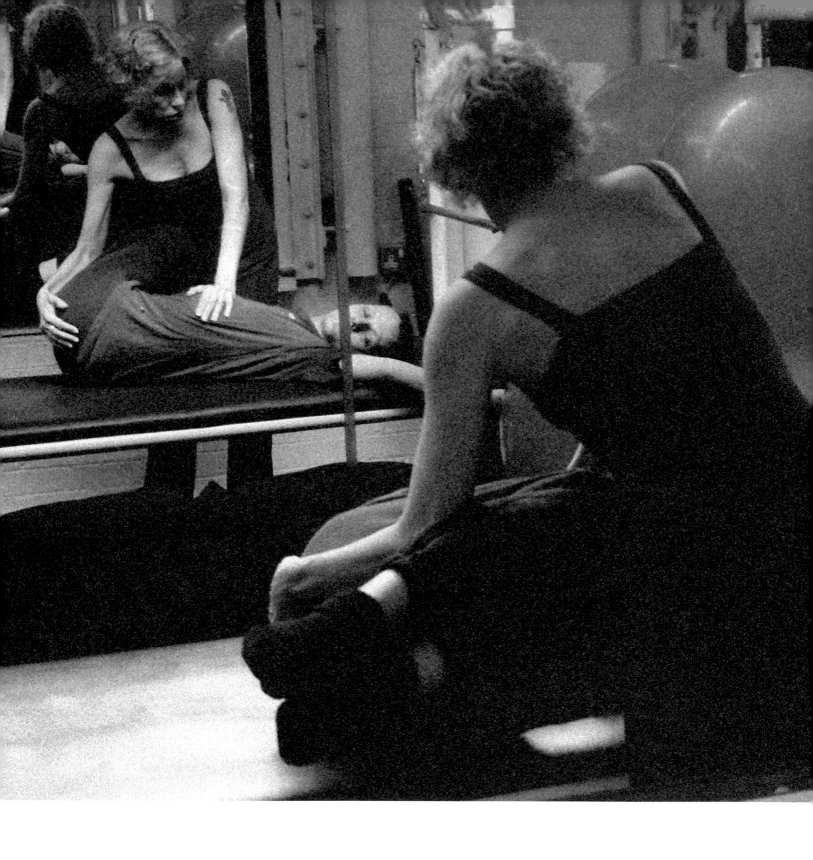

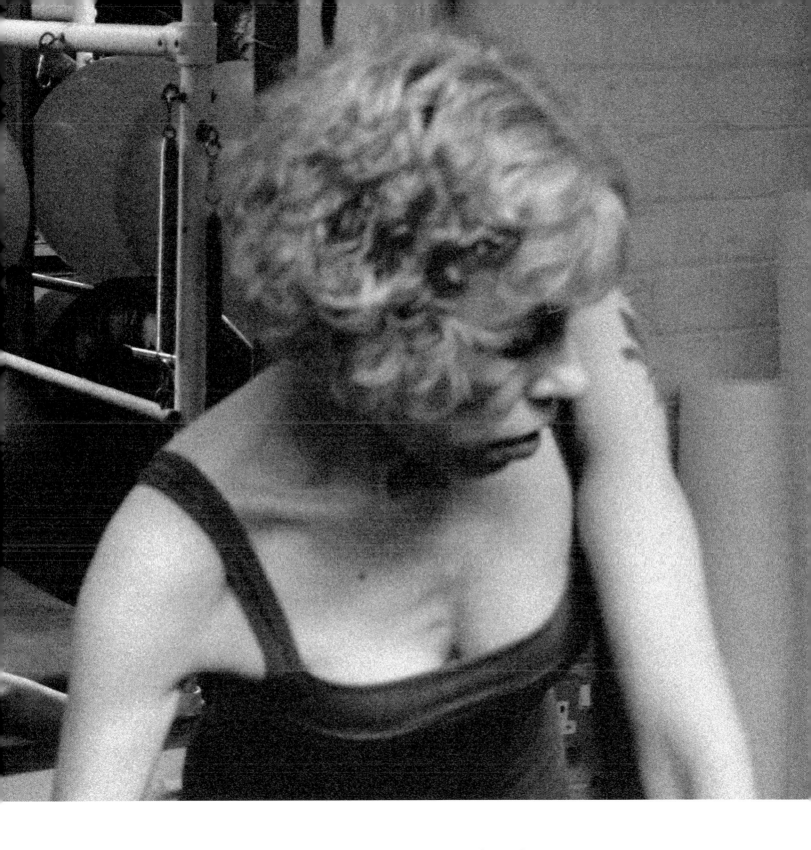

6 remedial exercises

For those of you who have any condition that affects muscles and joints, my Body Maintenance programme is a superb tool to use as you begin the journey towards helping and even reversing your condition. As previously stated, I absolutely believe everyone can and will improve, and even overcome, their physical difficulties with a safe and gentle group of exercises. You will be amazed at the body's ability to respond and rejuvenate, given the correct impetus. In this chapter are some specific exercises you can do every day to alleviate repetitive strain injury (carpal tunnel syndrome), scoliosis, sciatica or a bad back.

Note: The few remedial exercises contained in this book for each condition will not achieve the results possible in my studio and from individually taught programmes over an extended period of time.

BAD BACKS

The back causes more problems than almost any other part of the body. The spinal column provides support to the entire body and is the centre of all movement. The muscles in the back link the vertebrae of the spine to each other. It is not surprising, then, that if these muscles are weak or damaged through injury, all sorts of problems affecting alignment and stability may occur.

Muscular pain and stiffness in the joints can transpire for many different reasons, for example congenital conditions, injury, weak muscles, a slipped disc, etc. The shock-absorbing discs between the vertebrae may slip out of position and can damage the joints, leading to infections and degenerative problems. Pain varies depending on the cause of the problem and the person.

Conventional Treatment

Treatment may include anti-inflammatory drugs and painkillers, physiotherapy and surgery. Back problems can be notoriously difficult to eliminate.

Body Maintenance Method

Pilates-based exercises, as they focus on strengthening the muscles in the spine and abdomen, can be extremely beneficial for all sorts of back problems.

MORNING MAINTENANCE FOR BAD BACKS

This 10-minute exercise programme is based on the exercises many of my clients who have had back injuries or who suffer from chronic back pain do first thing in the morning. When you wake up in the morning with a bad back, you tend to feel quite immobile, stiff and uncomfortable. Your body doesn't want to move and you have difficulty even straightening up. This is a selection of six exercises to do in the morning between the time you get out of bed and go to work, which will strengthen and mobilize your lower back.

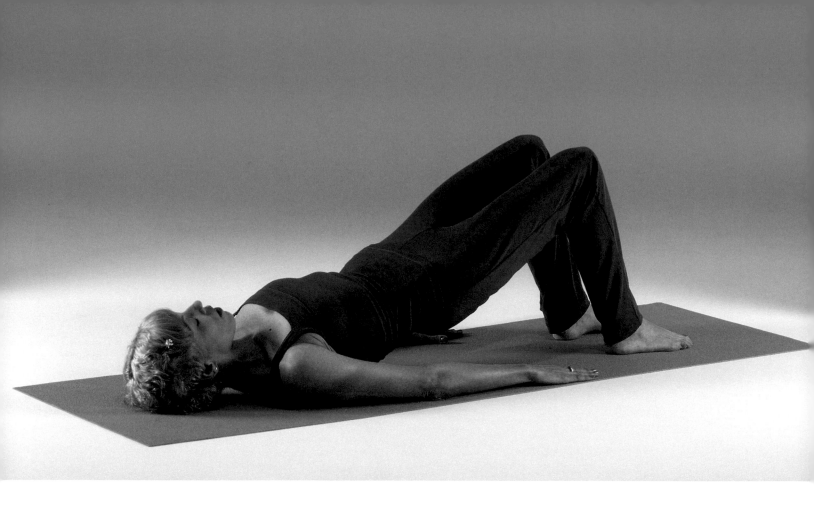

Pelvic Tilt

This is a basic pelvic tilt. (Compare page 44.) Lie on a towel or mat with your knees bent. You may also need to place a small towel behind your head. The feet, hips and knees are all parallel, hip-width apart; the tailbone is relaxed on the mat without feeling forced down. The shoulders are relaxed and the neck is long. The arms are softly beside you.

Without gripping your bottom, very gently tip your pelvis upwards as you breathe out, breathe in and lower. This is a low pelvic tilt. Don't lift higher than your waist. You are only lifting your lower back off the ground. It is important to exhale as you lift. Breathe in, keeping your neck long, and roll all the way down. Do approximately 10 repetitions.

Try to get that primary curve in your lower back working to warm up the lower back, bringing the blood supply into that area.

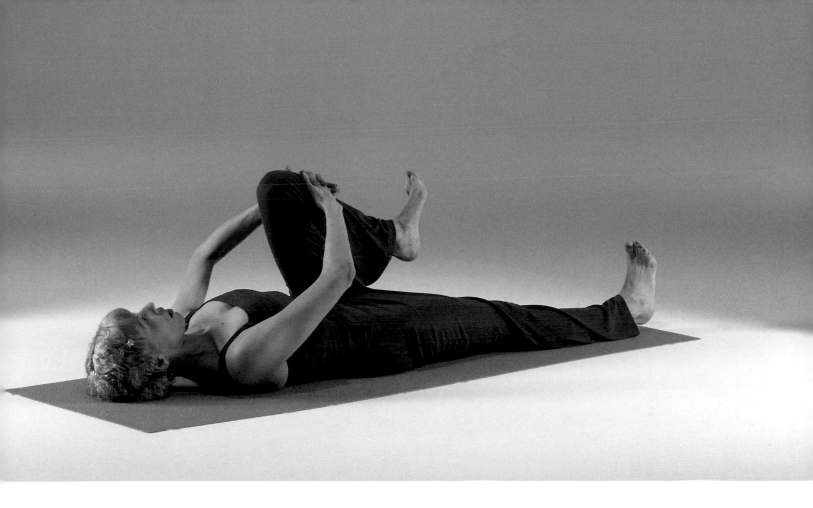

Passive Stretch for the Lower Back

Lie flat on the floor. This is a passive stretch for the lower back and the hamstrings. Very gently bend your right knee into your chest, holding on to the shin, below the kneecap. Have the elbows lifted to the side. You should not feel tension in your shoulders.

Breathe out and pull one knee into your chest, stretching the other leg along the floor and gently flexing both feet. You should feel a passive stretch going through the bent leg and buttock. You will also feel a hamstring and calf stretch going through the straight leg. Count: one, two, three, four. Then change sides. Do 10 repetitions altogether, alternating five on each leg.

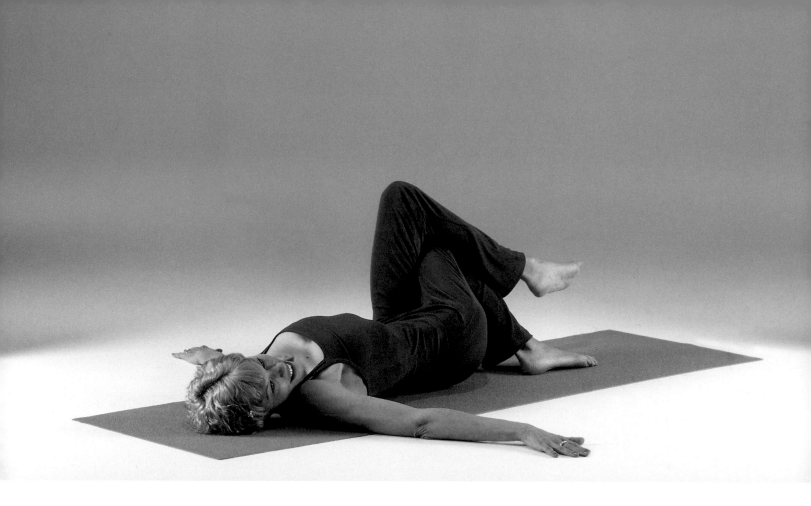

Hip Roll

This mobilization exercise for the spine will warm up the back. It is a gentle stretch for the lower back and the hip. The stomach is the instigator of the movement. You are in exactly the same position as for the pelvic tilt, but this time you cross one leg over the other. It doesn't matter which leg you start with, but the other foot is firmly on the floor.

The arms are beside you, palms facing down below shoulder level. The stomach is the stabilizer in this exercise, and at no point does either shoulder blade leave the mat.

Breathe in, breathe out and take a gentle twist one way, looking away from the direction you are twisting towards. Come back to the original position. Breathe in from the centre, and breathe out as you twist in the opposite direction.

You'll know if you've gone too far, as your stomach will protrude and your shoulders will leave the mat. If it's too hard for you to move your head and look in the opposite direction due to coordination problems, start by looking directly up while you familiarize yourself with the exercise. When you're comfortable you can begin turning the head.

Do 10 twists with one leg on top, then 10 twists with the other.

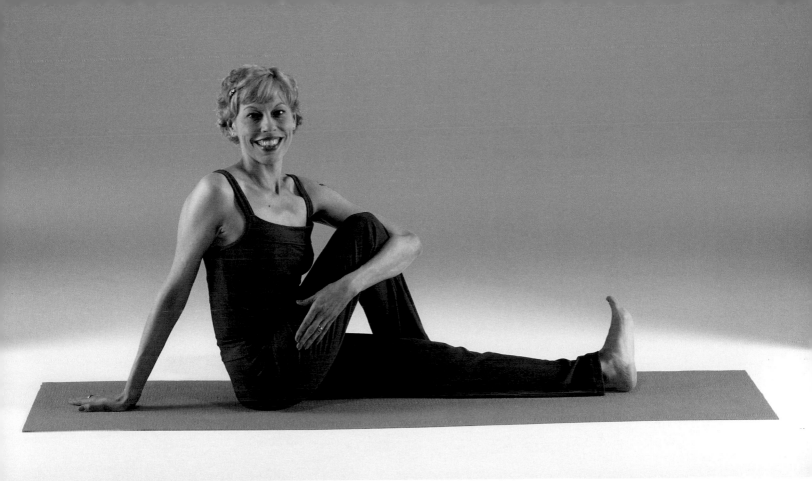

Basic Back of the Hip and Bottom Stretch

If you have a bad back, it is very likely that your buttock muscles and hamstrings will be tight. Sit on the floor, or lean against a wall.

Stretch your left leg out in front of you. Cross your right foot over your left knee, keeping your right hand on the floor. Hold on to your right knee with your left hand, as you gently ease that knee into your chest. Then rotate your body around to the right. The left leg in front of you is parallel to the floor. Keep your foot to the ceiling and your shoulders relaxed. Don't let your foot roll out of line with the knee. Feel the stretch through your buttock.

Repeat four times, each time alternating legs and the direction you turn. Hold each stretch for 30 seconds.

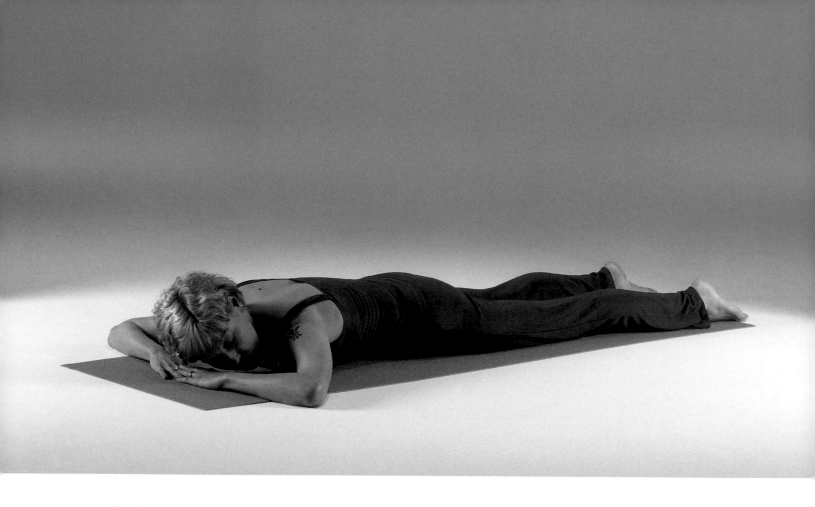

Basic Back Exercise

Lie face down, stomach on the floor. Relax your head to the side. Gently breathe in, and feel your stomach drop to the floor. Breathe out and pull your stomach into your spine so that your tailbone drops. Don't grip your bottom or tense your shoulders. Eventually you will be able to get your fingers in between your stomach and the floor as you breathe out. Feel your stomach working and your back strengthening. Both hip bones stay on the floor. Repeat 10 times.

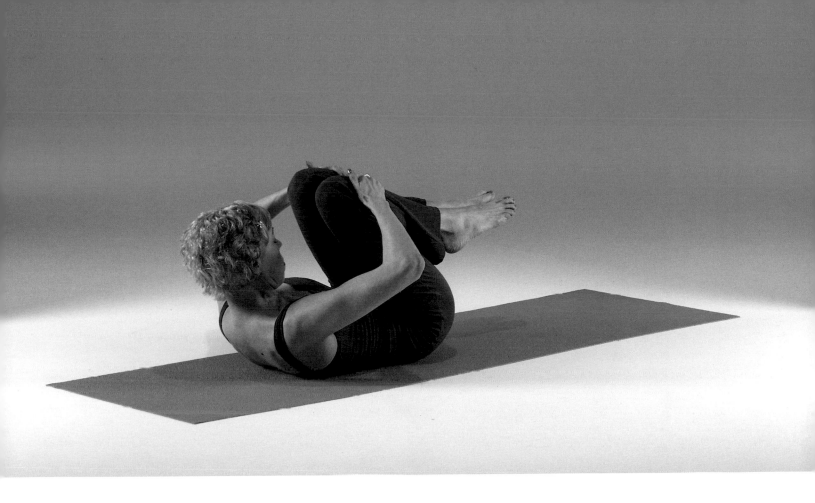

Spine Release Exercise

Roll over onto your back. Breathe in, then very gently
breathe out and, bending both knees to your chest, curl
your head towards your knees. Hold, breathe in, then
breathe out, and relax your head down, pulling your
stomach into your spine. This is a passive back and neck
stretch to stretch out your back. Do 10 repetitions.

WATCHPOINT

▷ Don't tense your shoulders; keep your bottom on
the floor.

SCIATICA

Sciatica is a radiating pain along the distribution of the sciatic nerve, which affects the buttocks and backs of the legs. It frequently causes pain in the lower back, or lumbago. In severe cases it may spread to the calf. The most common cause of sciatica is from a prolapsed intervertebral disc. This causes pressure on one or more of the nerve roots that originate in the lower part of the spinal cord and make up the sciatic nerve. Sciatica may also occur for a number of other reasons. For example, this condition may happen suddenly when a person is lifting something heavy. The amount of pain varies, depending on which nerve roots are affected, and ranges from mild discomfort to acute pain.

Conventional Treatment

The first course of action is usually a few weeks of bed rest. Sometimes sufferers are prescribed a spinal support or corset. If there is no improvement, the next step may involve surgery in order to remove the compression of the disc on the nerve root.

Body Maintenance Method

Pilates-based exercises can do much to alleviate this debilitating condition.

Back Strengthening

See page 62

Basic Back of Hip and Bottom Stretch

See page 153

Basic Back Exercise

See page 154

REPETITIVE STRAIN INJURY (CARPAL TUNNEL SYNDROME)

This is a common problem amongst people whose work involves some kind of repetitive action, such as typing at a keyboard all day or playing a musical instrument. There are various types of injury that can be sustained in the muscles, tendons and ligaments in the hands and wrists from repetitive motions. The most common is the compression of the median nerve as it passes under the ligament that lies across the front of the wrist.

Symptoms appear after prolonged activity, and include tingling and weakness or numbness in the fingers and hands. Sufferers may also experience aching, burning or shooting pains in the wrists and hands, which frequently spread to the forearms, neck, shoulders, upper back and upper arms. These symptoms get progressively worse until the person is barely able to use his or her hands at all, as the weakness makes it almost impossible to grasp objects properly. In the most severe cases the fingers may also swell up

Conventional Treatment

Anti-inflammatory drugs, which may be prescribed to reduce the inflammation and swelling, aren't always effective. Painkillers can obviously help to relieve the pain, and wearing a splint can immobilize the wrist and alleviate discomfort.

Sufferers find that symptoms can come and go over the years. If the condition is not treated, the pain may become intolerable. Some people have to resort to surgery, which involves making an incision from the anterior of the wrist to the palm of the hand. The surgical effects are variable and symptoms may continue afterwards

Body Maintentance Method

I have seen many people make a good recovery using the specific exercises I have evolved to treat this condition. These exercises are very gentle. They are designed to strengthen the hands and wrists and should be practised daily. As the hands and wrists get stronger and begin to regain proper mobility through exercise, the symptoms may disappear.

Wrist Strengthening

Holding onto your wrist with the other hand, make a fist with your hand. The wrist is in neutral. Gently lower your wrist down halfway, then bring it back to neutral again. Think of this as a resistance exercise. Imagine you're resisting very slowly. You can also do this with your hand facing up. Repeat 10 times.

You can do this using a small weight too (e.g., a tin of beans), but not if you feel any pain.

Wrist Circles

Holding onto your wrist with the other hand, circle the wrist slowly one way, and then the other. Repeat 10 times, then change hands.

WATCHPOINT

▷ If you're doing these exercises correctly your hands and wrists will feel warmer.

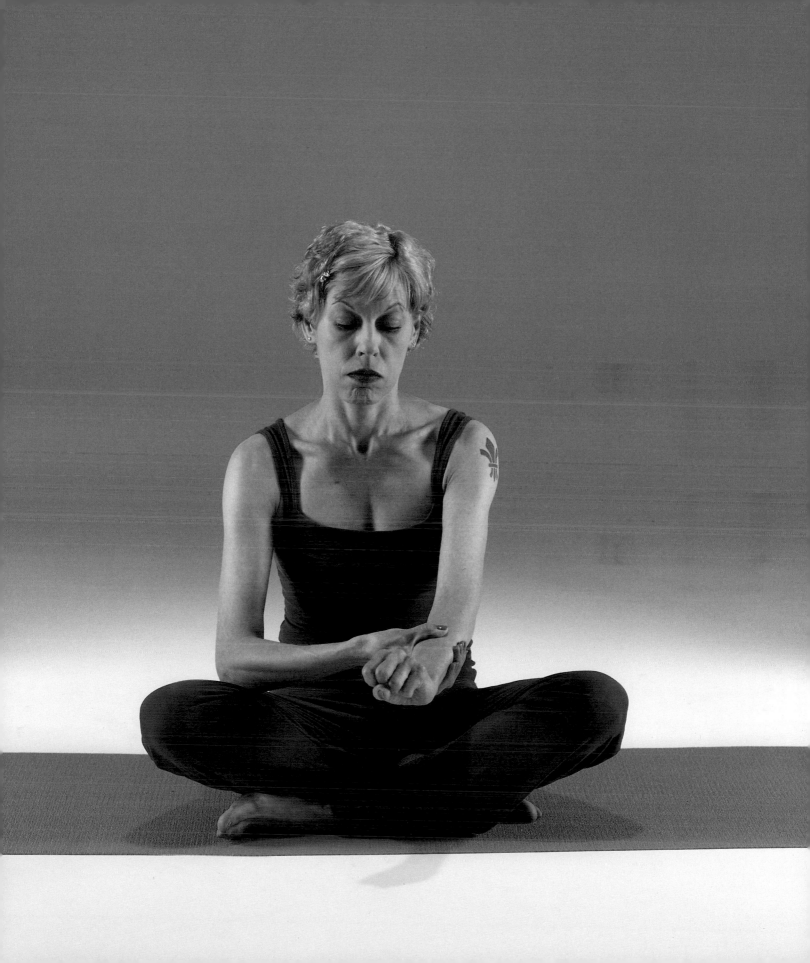

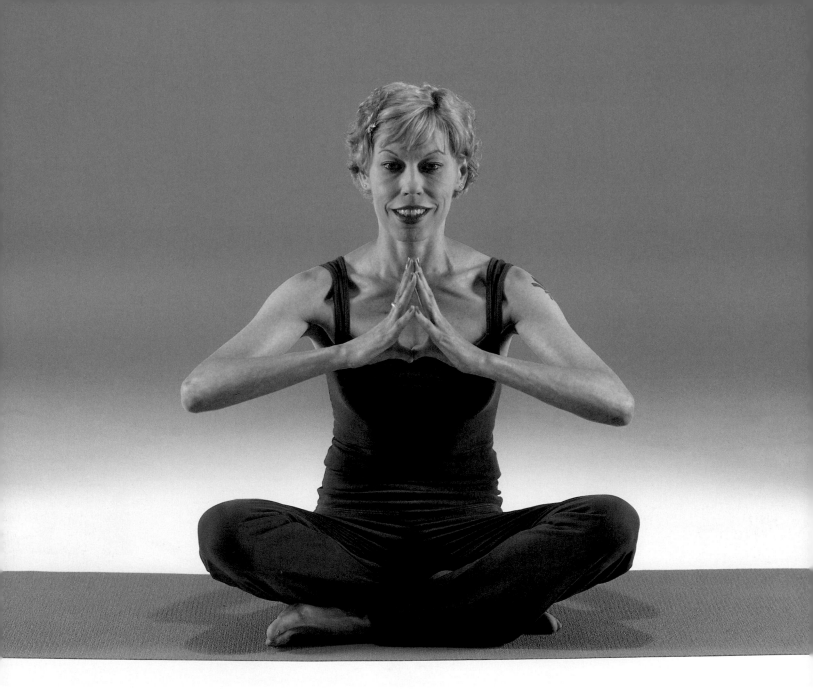

Hand and Finger Stretch

Place your hands so that the tips of the fingers and thumbs are touching. Imagine you're holding a soft ball. Press and resist your fingers – your hands don't close. Keep your shoulders relaxed and hands level with your chest. Relax and repeat 10 times.

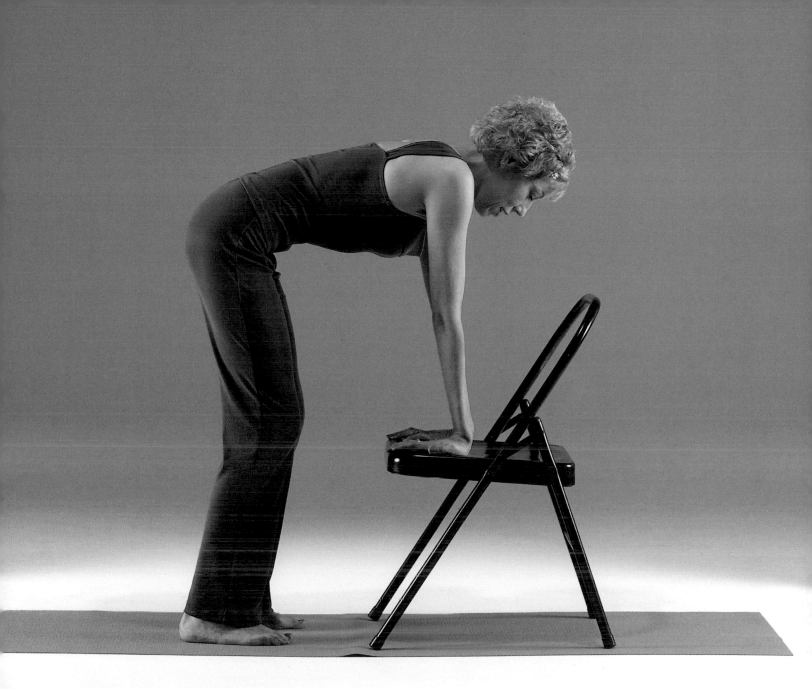

Wrist Stretch

Using a chair, place your hands on the seat, fingers towards you. Keep your elbows unlocked and gently lean your wrists into the chair. Don't press with your whole weight. Repeat four times. Shake your hands afterwards. Remember: don't lean too hard into the stretch.

SCOLIOSIS

Scoliosis is an extremely distressing condition that generates an S-shaped curvature of the spine. This is caused by a twist in the spine, which lead to the vertebrae becoming compressed and tilting to one side. In time this pressure can bring about fused vertebrae. Symptoms vary depending on the degree of the twist. There is generally a great deal of distress as the body struggles to accommodate this spinal imbalance, which forces the surrounding muscles into painful contortions.

Mild scoliosis may be barely noticeable, but in severe cases it leads to the formation of an unsightly hump and causes constant stooping, as the person is unable to stand upright. Scoliosis tends to first appear in adolescence and from then on, unless it is corrected while the body is still young and malleable, gets progressively worse.

Conventional Treatment

Treatment is usually very difficult. The most likely options for the scoliosis sufferer range from physiotherapy to surgical intervention. There are now several complex types of operations to try and correct it, or at least prevent the condition from worsening. However, these are not always successful.

Body Maintenance Method

I have devised a number of exercises designed to build up the weak muscles in the back and uncurl the spine, and have been witness to some remarkable changes.

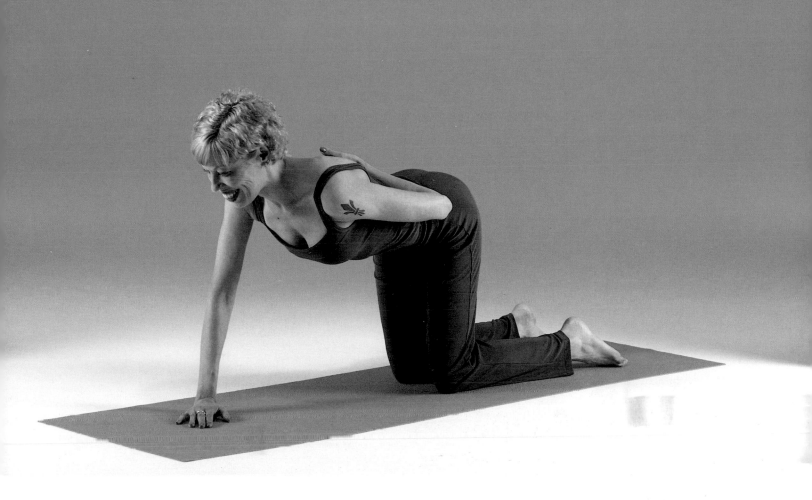

WATCHPOINTS

▷ Don't lock your elbows.

▷ Don't lift your head too high or you may strain your neck.

▷ As you press your chest down to the floor in the reverse exercise, if you feel any pinching in your lower back you've gone too far.

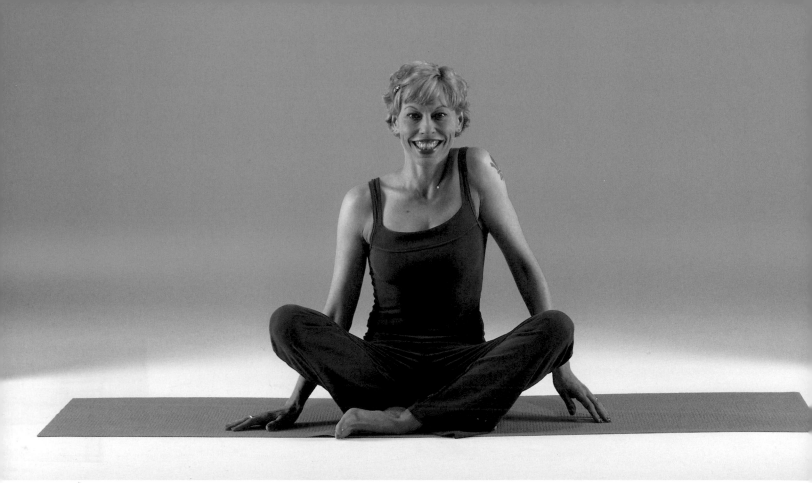

The following three exercises can either be done on the floor, or sitting on a chair.

Single Shoulder Lifts

These work the shoulder joints and blades.

Sit comfortably. Breathe in, and slowly squeeze your right shoulder up to your right ear. Relax it down. Repeat with other shoulder. Do this to a count of four up, four down. Don't move your head. Repeat 10 times, alternating shoulders.

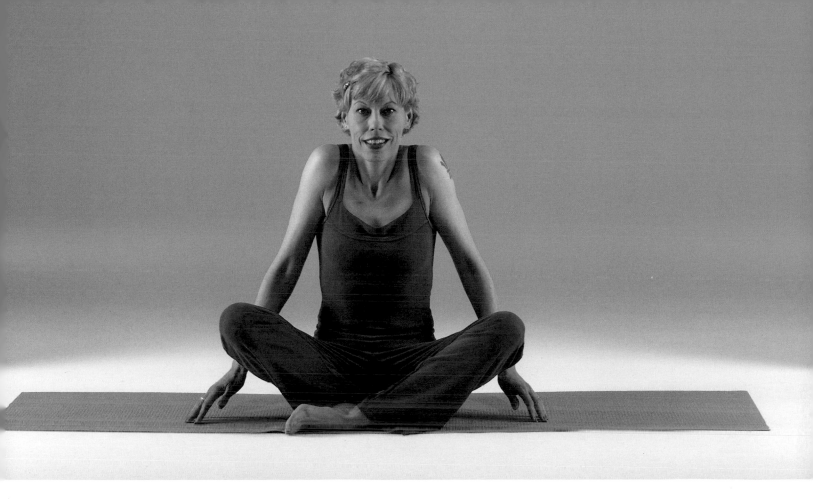

Double Shoulder Lifts

Sitting as above, squeeze both shoulders up to your ears.
Make sure your hands are dangling loosely by your sides.
If you feel you are arching your back, use a wall as
support. Repeat 10 times.

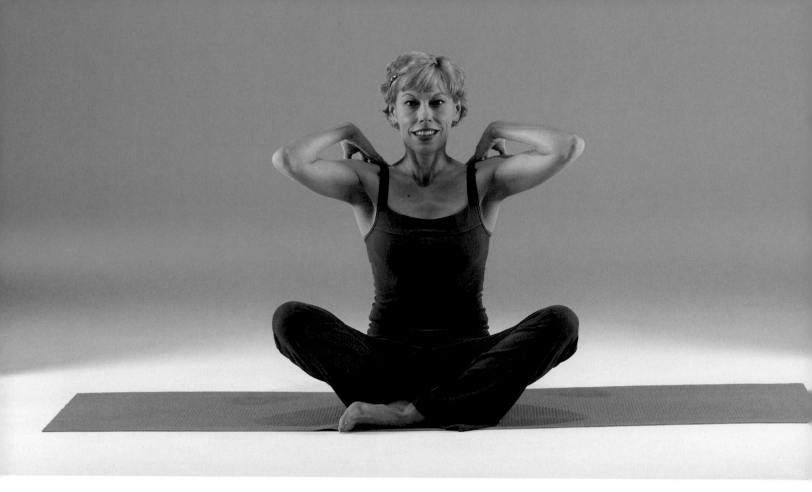

Shoulder Circles

Assume the same position as above. With both your hands on your shoulders, very gently circle both arms forward. Repeat 10 times. Then circle your arms backwards and again, repeat 10 times. If this feels uncomfortable, circle your shoulders with your arms at your sides.

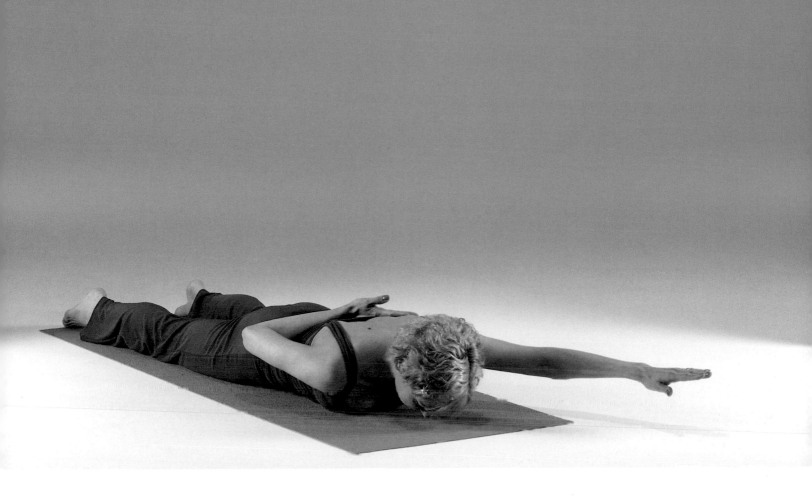

Single Arm Stretch

Lie on your stomach and imagine you're a small starfish.
Your arms are slightly wider than your shoulders, your
forehead on the floor on a folded towel. Make sure your
legs are comfortably apart and rotated slightly outwards.
Place your right arm on your back reaching towards the
left shoulder blade. Breathe out and let your left arm
gently float off the ground. As your arm reaches away,
think of your shoulder blade 'gliding'. You should feel this
with the hand on your back. Make sure that as your
stomach goes in, your pelvis drops. As you breathe out,
don't grip your bottom.

   Repeat four times, first on one side then the other.
Then go into the relaxation position (see page 69).

The following exercises are done against a wall. These will help to stretch out the shoulder blades and the upper back.

Arm Stretch Against the Wall

Stand sideways on to a wall, about a foot away from it. Place your hand palm down on the wall. Do not arch your back. Very gently slide up the wall, leaning your body weight in to your palm, stretching your shoulder. Don't let the hips shift. Hold for a few seconds. Repeat four to six times, changing sides each time.

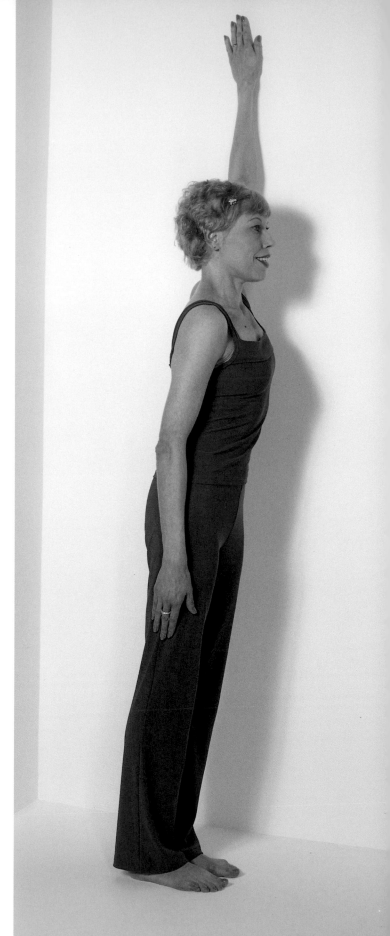

Arm Stretch Against the Wall 2

Stand facing the wall, with one hand on top of the other
against it Keep your stomach in, tailbone dropped. Don't
stick your bottom out. Gently stretch up the wall. Hold for
a few seconds. Repeat 10 times, changing the hand on top.

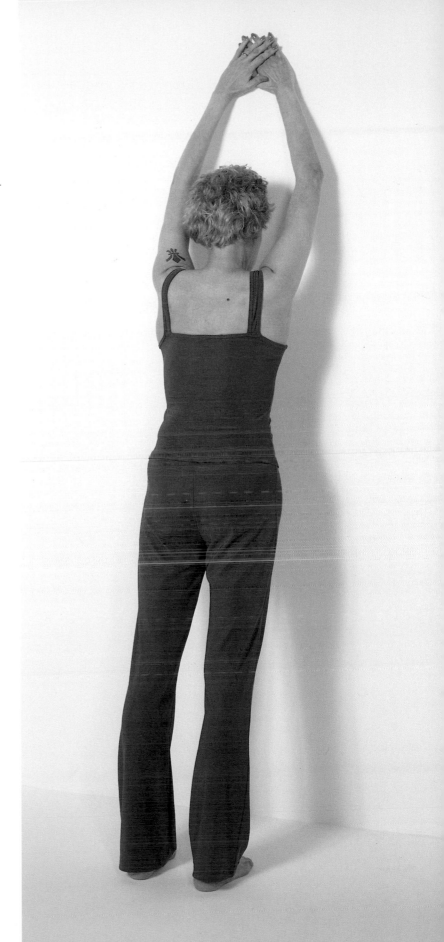

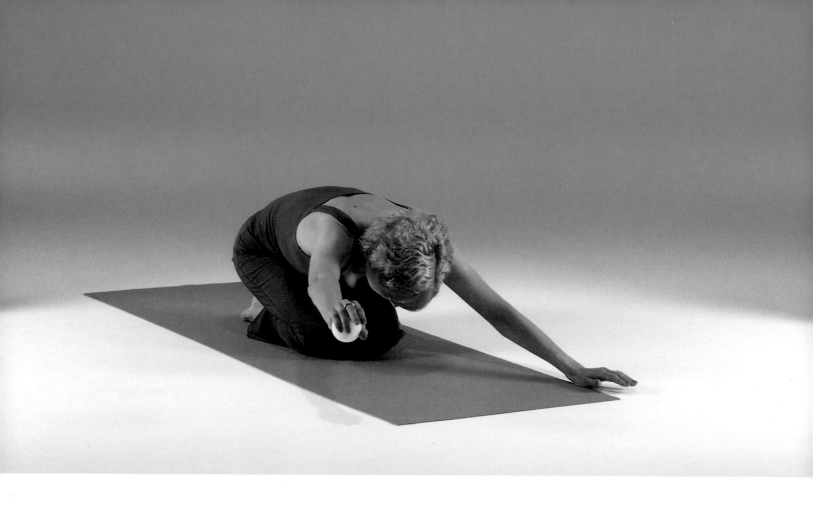

The following two exercises are done kneeling on the floor. However, if you find this too difficult, you can sit on a chair and use a table to do them. You can do them either with or without the tennis ball.

Alternate Arm Lift

To work the shoulders and shoulder blades.

Sit down on your heels in the relaxation position (see page 69). Have both hands wider than the shoulders and keep your head relaxed. Take a tennis ball in one hand and slowly, without moving anything else, lift that hand off the floor. Hold for a few seconds and relax back down. Don't twist your body or lift your head. You should feel your shoulder doing all the work. Change hands and repeat up to 10 times.

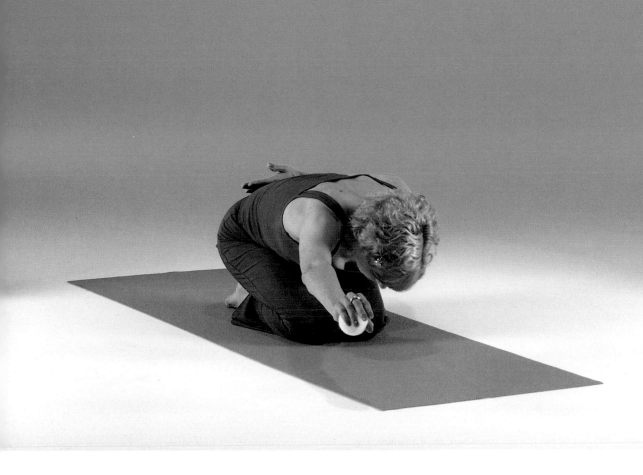

Alternate Arm Lift 2

Assume the same position as in the previous exercise.
This time, keep the hand that you are not lifting behind
your back.

CONCLUSION

The benefits of embarking on this exercise programme are manifold. As in any DIY book, until you familiarize yourself with all the material and go through it at your own pace, it may seem a bit confusing. You will find that once you coordinate your movements with the correct breathing any apprehension will soon vanish.

While the material is still fresh, before you close this book, why not try some of the simple visualization exercises right now? Close your eyes – scan your body – visit each area. What do you feel? Is any area painful or weak? Do you immediately focus on one area? Try some of the simple postural exercises to get a feeling of alignment. Imagine how you wish to appear.

Your body represents the sum of its parts – therefore each part must be fully conversant with the others. Fluency can be achieved by allowing the mind–body–spirit connection to evolve. This is a challenge that can be met with calm determination and a vision of purpose.

Everybody's potential is limitless. We can look forward to ageing well, living longer and having more productive lives. We often pay no attention to our bodies until something goes wrong. The human body is a splendid vehicle. In addition to our physical beings, it houses our emotional and spiritual selves. Like a car, it requires regular maintenance, especially since it can't be traded in. Our bodies remain with us all our lives. It is not costly or painful to respect and maintain them.
With Body Maintenance you can slowly recreate a sense of physical vitality and core stability, and look forward to continued well-being and health.

You now have the tools. Good luck!

INDEX

hamstring toner and
strengthener 76
lying hamstring stretch 90–1
standing hamstring stretch
88–9
hand exercises 142–3
hand and finger stretch 160
Herdman, Alan 5
hips
exercises
back and hip – gluteal stretch
81
back and hip - gluteal stretch
(2) 82
back of the hip and bottom
stretch, basic 153, 156
hip flexor and front of thigh
exercise 94–5
hip mobility exercise 116–19
hip roll 152
muscles 80
HIV related problems 5
holistic approach viii
hyperextension 21

I

imbalances, in the body 2
inhaling 16
internal oblique (muscle) 26
inversion 22

K

key terms 19–26

L

latissimus dorsi (muscle) 24, 25, 26
lat exercise 102–3
legs
exercises 70, 80
back and hip – gluteal stretch
81
back and hip – gluteal stretch
(2) 82
bottom toner 77
bottom toner (2) 78
bottom toner (3) 79
hamstring toner and
strengthener 76
hip flexor and front of thigh
exercise 94–5
inner thigh stretch 92
inner thigh stretch, advanced
93
inside thigh circles 72
inside thigh lift 71
lying calf stretch 86–7
lying hamstring stretch 90–1
outer thigh lift 73
outer thighs and buttocks 74
outer thighs and buttocks (2)
75
quadriceps stretch 83
quadriceps stretch, advanced
84–5
quadriceps stretch, advanced
(2) 86
standing calf stretch 88
standing hamstring stretch
88–9
muscles 5, 36
relaxing 20

lengthening the body viii, 11
levator scapulae (muscle) 23, 24, 25
lower body (legs hips and thighs) x
lumbago 156
lumbar vertebrae 21, 22

M

mat exercises, functions of 5
mats, exercise 113
medical conditions viii, x, 2–3, 31, 32,
36, 148, 156–7, 162
mental improvement 5
midday break exercises 136
calf stretch 138–9
cat stretch at the desk (shoulders)
144
doming feet 137
hand exercises 142–3
shoulder rotation 140–1
shoulder stretch 138–9, 145
mind
focusing ix
mind and body integration 4, 5,
8–12, 18, 174
mindful exercise 9–10
over matter 8
morning energizing exercises 113
full-body wake-up stretch 120
hip mobility exercise 116–19
waist stretch 124–5
warm-ups for shoulder and back 121
movements 21, 23
muscles 21, 23, 24–5, 26
'antagonistic pairs' 23
strengthening 2, 5, 11
stretching tight 2, 11

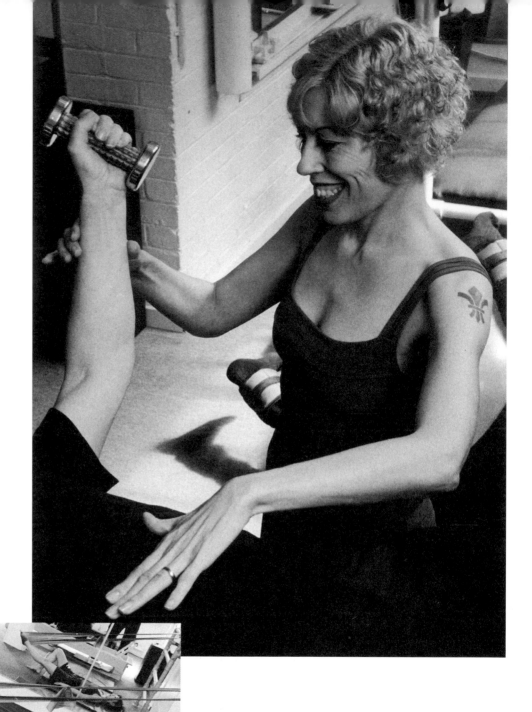

For further information on The Body Maintenance Studio
please send a stamped addressed envelope to:
Body Maintenance Studio
2nd Floor
Pineapple
7 Langley Street
London WC2H 9JA